Student Workbook to Accompany
Fundamental Orthopedic
Management for the
Physical Therapist Assistant

Student Workbook to Accompany Fundamental Orthopedic Management for the Physical Therapist Assistant

Gary A. Shankman, PTA

NovaCare
Atlanta, Georgia

with 44 illustrations

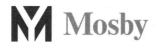 Mosby

St. Louis Baltimore Boston Carlsbad Chicago Naples New York Philadelphia Portland
London Madrid Mexico City Singapore Sydney Tokyo Toronto Wiesbaden

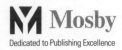

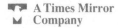

Publisher: Don Ladig
Executive Editor: Martha Sasser
Developmental Editor: Kellie F. White
Editorial Assistant: Laura A. MacAdam
Project Manager: Mark Spann
Production Editors: Jennifer Doll, Julie Eddy
Designer: Jeanne Wolfgeher
Manufacturing Supervisor: Tony McAllister

Printed in the United States of America
Composition by Carlisle Communications, Ltd.
Printing/binding by R.R. Donnelley & Sons Company

Mosby-Year Book, Inc.
11830 Westline Industrial Drive
St. Louis, Missouri 63146

ISBN 0-8151-7542-6

97 98 99 00 01 / 9 8 7 6 5 4 3 2 1

*To my wife Judy,
and my sons,
Kyle, Tyler, and Jordan.*

Preface

This study guide is designed to test retention, to support current practical and purposeful understanding of the fundamental principles of clinical orthopedic physical therapy, and to challenge the student's ability to apply basic concepts through the process of critical thinking and analysis.

Developed to accompany the text *Fundamental Orthopedic Management for the Physical Therapist Assistant,* this testing instrument is organized in sequential fashion, whereby basic concepts lead to analytical, creative application of theory and problem solving. The design method used to develop this study guide, therefore, lends itself to concept exploration, independent thinking, and student collaboration through critical thinking questions that foster interaction and stimulate comprehension of fundamental principles.

The challenge in creating this study guide was to identify and emphasize key teaching objectives that center on the evaluation of student comprehension and to ultimately demonstrate appropriate clinical application of various concepts, theories, and principles of orthopedic physical therapy practice.

This study guide includes multiple choice questions, short answer questions, fill-in statements, figure identification, labeling, true-false questions, and essay questions. In addition, critical thinking application questions provide an avenue for student collaboration, student-teacher interaction, group presentations, case study development, role playing, independent thinking, and various class activities.

Therefore, this study guide can accommodate a wide range of unique and creative teaching styles and will perhaps, most importantly, provide the student with a rewarding learning experience.

Contents

Basic Concepts of Orthopedic Management

Patient Supervision and Observation During Treatment

KEY TERMS

Responsibility
Communication
Listening
Accountability
Proactive
Probing questions
Open-end questions
Closed-end questions
Dominance
Submission
Hostility
Warmth
Basic dimensional model
Recognition

MULTIPLE CHOICE

1. Throughout patient supervision and observation, the physical therapist assistant will:
   A. Observe the patient and note any and all changes in objective clinical data
   B. Provide intermittent supervision throughout treatment
   C. Assess changes noted in initial clinical data obtained by the physical therapist and immediately alter the treatment program prior to consultation with the physical therapist
   D. Constantly interact, observe, and supervise each patient, comparing initial clinical evaluation data with any changes noted in the patient's condition, then reporting these changes to the supervising therapist prior to altering the treatment program

E. A, B, and C
F. A and D

SHORT ANSWER

2. List five components of patient supervision.
3. Identify six members of the rehabilitation team who also may be involved with patient supervision.
4. Effective _____ is the hallmark of a great team and should be maximized.
5. Appropriate medical language used with the patient and his or her family helps to convey _____ , _____ , _____ , and _____ .
6. The physical therapist assistant must also be aware that _____ is an effective communication tool.
7. Which type of probing questions invites the patient to share feelings, thoughts, and opinions?
8. Which type of probing questions is directed toward finding facts, obtaining specific responses, and filling in details?
9. Give three examples of open-end probing questions that may be appropriate during the course of patient observation and interactive supervision.
10. Give three examples of closed-end probing questions that may be appropriate during the course of patient observation and interactive supervision.
11. Which type of statements checks understanding, helps patients clarify thinking, and provides direction for the clinician?
12. Give two examples of summary-type statements.
13. Identify four categories of human behavior as described by Buzzotta and Lefton.
14. In the following figure, label and identify the components of the dimensional model and the quadrants formed by combining two dimensions.

21. Discuss the skills required to provide patient supervision.
22. Define objective scales of measurements used to communicate changes in a patient's status to the physical therapist.
23. Apply proactive listening skills and objective scales of measurement to provide appropriate, accountable, and responsible observation and supervision of the patient during treatment.
24. Define open-end and closed-end questioning.
25. Define the quadrants of the basic dimensional model.
26. Discuss the four categories of behavior: dominance, submission, hostility, and warmth.
27. Describe the differences between "prompting" and "cueing."

CRITICAL THINKING APPLICATION

As a role-playing activity, one student will act the part of a patient, and another student will play the role of a practicing PTA. Using the dimensional model as a guide, the PTA should demonstrate proactive, participatory supervision skills, using appropriate probing questions and behavior consistent with the Q4 quadrant. Guide the patient in developing open-end questions, closed-end questions, and summary statements to convey compassion, understanding, interest, focus, and task specific actions to clarify and enhance the effectiveness of treatment.

The students will switch roles and the student now playing the PTA will use behaviors consistent with Q1, Q2, and Q3 quadrants of the dimensional model. Compare the effectiveness of using Q4 behavior with patient supervision with that of Q1, Q2, and Q3.

If you were a patient, how would you prefer to be treated? Which supervisory skills convey trust? Which behavior would you, as a patient, expect from the PTA?

15. Applying the dimensional model to the use of open-end and closed-end probing questions, which quadrant would represent the behavioral goal of the physical therapist assistant during patient supervision?
16. List seven qualities that are found in Q4 behavior.
17. Give an example of "prompting" a patient to attempt a specific task.
18. Give an example of "cueing" a patient to attempt a specific task.
19. Give nine examples of objective, measurable data that can help guide the assistant and supervising physical therapist to make appropriate modifications in a patient's treatment.

ESSAY QUESTIONS

Answer on a separate sheet of paper.
20. Identify and discuss the rationale for clear and concise communication among all members of the rehabilitation team.

Flexibility

KEY TERMS

Flexibility
Range of motion (ROM)
Collagen
Stress
Strain
Elastic deformation
Plastic deformation
Static stretching
Ballistic stretching
Proprioceptive neuromuscular facilitation (PNF)
Specificity
Golgi tendon organs (GTO)
Muscle spindles
Scar tissue
Contracture
Adhesions
Low-load, prolonged stretch

MULTIPLE CHOICE

1. Two components of flexibility are:
   A. Speed and joint motion
   B. Tension and stretch
   C. Elongation of muscle and range of motion
   D. Range of motion and tension
2. Collagen is a:
   A. Muscle
   B. Protein
   C. Mucopolysaccharide
   D. Carbohydrate
3. Collagen is found in:
   A. Muscle
   B. Bone

C. Tendon
D. Capsule
E. All of the above
4. The most common types of collagen found in joint capsule and muscle are:
   A. Types I and II
   B. Types III and IV
   C. Types I and III
   D. Types II and III
5. *Strain* is defined as:
   A. Too much stress
   B. Tearing of tissue
   C. Painful stretching
   D. Proportional elongation of tissue during stress
   E. All of the above
6. Two viscoelastic properties of connective tissue are:
   A. Stress and strain
   B. Rate and tension
   C. Plastic and elastic deformation
   D. Speed and tissue failure
7. Goals of static stretching are:
   A. To improve athletic performance
   B. To increase ligament stability
   C. To reduce contractures; improve motion; minimize risk of soft tissue injury
   D. To decrease muscle tension
   E. All of the above
8. A general body warmup preceding ballistic stretching or static stretching helps to: (circle any that apply)
   A. Teach the patient proper form
   B. Duplicate ADLs
   C. Increase tissue temperature
   D. Reduce risk of connective tissue damage
   E. Improve sports performance

9. A permanent or transient limitation of movement or shortening of muscle or other soft tissue is called:
   A. Scar tissue
   B. Joint adhesion
   C. Rupture
   D. Contracture

10. A limitation of function that results from the formation of scar tissue is called a(n):
    A. Nodule
    B. Adhesion
    C. Contracture
    D. None of the above

11. Long duration static stretching refers to holding the stretch for:
    A. 20 seconds
    B. 1 to 5 minutes
    C. 10 to 12 minutes
    D. 20 to 60 minutes

SHORT ANSWER

12. Muscle tissue is considered to be (*active* or *passive*) restraint to joint motion.
13. Name three types of active stretching.
14. A(n) _____ is an inhibitory neurophysiological sensory receptor involved with the stretch reflex.
15. The _____ is an excitatory specialized fiber found in muscle.

TRUE/FALSE

16. T or F Stress is the amount of tension or load placed on tissues.
17. T or F Tissue temperature does not affect connective tissue extensibility.
18. T or F Active exercise has an effect on intramuscular temperature and tissue extensibility.
19. T or F PNF stretching is superior to other forms of active stretching.
20. T or F Low-load, long-duration static stretching is a technique used to stretch soft tissue contractures.
21. T or F Scar tissue is strong and fully mature at 60 days following injury or surgical repair.
22. T or F To effectively stretch scar tissue, maximum stress must be applied.

ESSAY QUESTIONS

Answer on a separate sheet of paper.
23. Define and discuss range of motion and flexibility.
24. Identify the properties of connective tissue.
25. Explain the differences between stress and strain.
26. Describe plastic deformation and elastic deformation.
27. Discuss how temperature affects connective tissue.
28. Identify and describe various stretching techniques.
29. Define Golgi tendon organs (GTOs) and muscle spindles.
30. Describe the clinical applications for stretching soft tissue contractures.
31. Describe and contrast the differences and similarities between scar tissue and adhesions.
32. Outline various methods used to measure flexibility.

CRITICAL THINKING APPLICATION

In small groups, outline and thoroughly describe methods, techniques, and protocols to effectively treat a soft tissue knee flexion contracture. Which therapeutic agents would you recommend? For how long? Which specific stretching techniques would you use? Would strengthening play a part in overcoming the contracture during the flexibility program? How? Distinguish exactly what you are attempting to correct or enhance. How does scar tissue affect function? How do adhesions affect function? Organize your thoughts and discussion in an orderly, specific sequence that relates to immature and mature scar tissue and details which stretching techniques to use during various phases of recovery.

Contrast this discussion with techniques you would recommend for improving muscle extensibility in a patient who demonstrates tight hamstrings and complains of low back dysfunction. How does ballistic stretching play a role in your program? Does temperature affect soft tissue extensibility, and if so, how would you employ or recommend thermal agents in the treatment of tight hamstrings? Discuss specific examples of PNF stretching, static and ballistic stretching, and the application of each.

Strength

Epimysium
Fasciculus
Perimysium
Endomysium
Myofibrils
Actin
Myosin
Slow twitch (ST) (type I–red–oxidative) muscle fiber
Fast twitch (FT) (type II–white–glycolytic) muscle
   fiber
Concentric
Eccentric
Isometric
Strength
Tension
Work
Power
Hypertrophy
Atrophy
SAID principle
Delayed onset muscle soreness (DOMS)
Progressive resistance exercise (PRE)
Plyometrics
Closed kinetic chain exercise (CKC)

MULTIPLE CHOICE

1. An individual muscle's potential to gain strength
   and power is determined by:
   A. Muscle fiber length
   B. Mass of the muscle
   C. Angle of attachment of the muscle to a tendon
   D. All of the above

2. Red muscle fibers are also identified as:
   A. Slow twitch
   B. Type I fibers
   C. Oxidative
   D. All of the above
3. White muscle fibers: (circle any that apply)
   A. Have more mitochondria
   B. Contain succinic dehydrogenase
   C. Are larger in diameter than red fibers
   D. Have low myoglobin
   E. Are recruited for endurance activities
4. White, fast twitch, glycolytic type II muscle fiber
   can be further classified into how many subclassifi-
   cations?
   A. Two
   B. Three
   C. Five
   D. Four
   E. None of the above
5. Circle the examples of muscle contractions.
   A. Isotonic
   B. Concentric
   C. Isokinetic
   D. Eccentric
   E. Isometric
6. Which testing tool affords the clinician the greatest
   degree of evaluating muscular performance?
   A. Hand dynamometers
   B. Cable tensiometry
   C. One-repetition maximum lifts
   D. Isokinetics
7. The data collected from an isokinetic dynamometer
   measures:
   A. Strength (force)
   B. Torque
   C. Power

D. Work

E. All of the above

8. The foundations of all clinically applied strength programs involve which of the following principles? (circle any that apply)

A. Overload

B. Duration

C. Specificity

D. Reversibility

E. Order

9. To best stimulate type I fibers, which program would be most appropriate? (circle any that apply)

A. High intensity - short duration

B. Low intensity - long duration

C. Stationary cycle ergometer

D. Upper body ergometer

E. One repetition max on the leg press

10. High-intensity resistance exercise leads to increases in: (circle any that apply)

A. ATP

B. Creatine kinase

C. Creatine phosphate

D. Succinic dehydrogenase

E. Type I muscle fibers

11. Which of the following more accurately describe the symptoms of delayed onset muscle soreness (DOMS)? (circle any that apply)

A. Local muscle pain

B. Diffuse muscle soreness

C. Specific intense injury

D. General muscle soreness

E. Radiating pain

12. Which of the following muscle contraction types result in the greatest occurrence of DOMS?

A. Isometric

B. Eccentric

C. Concentric

D. Isokinetic

E. Isotonic

13. When full arc motions of slow-speed, high-resistance exercise are used to generate greater tension and strength, the joint compression forces and resultant torque will be:

A. Reduced

B. The same as with high-speed, low-resistance exercise

C. Increased

D. Greatly reduced

14. To minimize joint compression forces during the initial stages of recovery, the most appropriate muscle contraction to use to develop or maintain strength would be:

A. Short arc eccentrics

B. Isokinetic full arc high-speed concentric

C. Isometrics

D. Slow-speed short arc isokinetic concentric

15. The angular velocity of the human knee during normal walking is approximately:

A. 60 degrees per second

B. 240 degrees per second

C. 180 degrees per second

D. 200 degrees per second

16. To recover functional use of the knee following injury, which of the following best describes the most appropriate selection of muscle contraction types to regain strength?

A. Isometrics - isotonic (concentric)

B. Isometrics - isotonic (eccentric)

C. Isometrics - isotonic (concentric and eccentric)

D. Isotonic (concentric and eccentric) - isokinetic slow speed (concentric and eccentric)

17. High velocity isokinetic exercise can allow for:

A. Accommodation of the patient's pain

B. Reduced compression forces

C. Improved functional speeds of contraction

D. All of the above

18. Which PRE program does the following describe: three sets of 10 repetitions of exercises, with the first set performed at 50% of 10 RM, the second set at 75% of 10 RM, and the third set at 100% of 10 RM?

A. Oxford

B. Regressive resistance exercise program

C. DeLorme PRE

D. DAPRE

19. Which of the following describes the rule of tens when applied to isometric exercise?

A. 10 body parts must be exercised

B. 10 exercises must be used

C. 10-second contractions, 10 repetitions, 10-second rest

D. None of the above

20. When instructing a patient to perform isometric contractions, which of the following best describes the most appropriate sequence?

A. 8-second contraction, 2-second rest

B. 10-second maximal contraction

C. 5-second contraction, 5-second rest

D. Gradual 2-second development of tension, 6-second maintenance of maximum contraction, gradual 2-second decrease in tension

21. Which of the following best describes an open kinetic chain (OKC)?

A. Wall squats

B. Supine leg press

C. Biceps curls

D. Stair steppers

22. A closed kinetic chain (CKC) exercise for the knee would be:

A. Short arc quads

B. Isometric quad sets

C. Seated knee extension

D. Supine leg press

E. All of the above

23. Climbing stairs is an example of:

A. Open kinetic chain exercise

B. Closed kinetic chain exercise

C. Open and closed chain exercise

D. Plyometric exercise

E. All of the above

24. The general rationale for utilizing CKC exercises in rehabilitation is:

A. To improve neuromuscular coordination

B. To stimulate muscular co-contractions

C. Joint approximation leads to increases in kinesthetic awareness

D. CKC exercises are more functional than OKC exercises

E. All of the above

SHORT ANSWER

25. How many muscle fiber types have been identified in humans?

26. Aerobic exercises require muscle fibers that are primarily _____ . (*oxidative* or *glycolytic*)

27. Organize the following five muscle fiber types into a numeric sequence of recruitment, proceeding from the lowest force requirements (1) to the greatest (5):

___ Fast twitch (type II)

___ Fast twitch (type II-AB)

___ Slow twitch (type I)

___ Fast twitch (type II-A)

___ Fast twitch (type II-B)

28. List the five ways muscular strength is measured.

29. Organize the following muscle contraction types in orderly sequence from greatest (3) to least (1) use of ATP.

___ Eccentrics

___ Concentrics

___ Isometrics

30. Organize the following muscle contraction types in orderly sequence from greatest (3) to least (1) force production.

___ Concentrics

___ Isometrics

___ Eccentrics

31. Name the two categories of muscle mutability.

32. What does *SAID* stand for?

33. Name the three stimuli for adaptive changes in skeletal muscles.

34. A patient returns to the outpatient physical therapy department and reports localized, specific muscle pain and describes an isolated event of lifting a box, which immediately increased pain. Describe the appropriate course of action the PTA will take to manage this patient's complaints of increased pain.

TRUE/FALSE

35. T or F   *Isokinetic* and *isotonic* do not describe muscle contractions but rather are terms used to define and describe events utilizing true muscle contractions.

36. T or F   Manual muscle testing can be used to determine a muscle's power, work capacity, and force production.

37. T or F   Clinically it is important to choose one contraction type throughout the course of recovery from injury.

38. T or F   In terms of muscle hypertrophy, type I fibers hypertrophy more than type II fibers.

39. T or F   Stretching an innervated muscle creates tension, which results in muscle hypertrophy.

40. T or F   Muscle soreness is never an anticipated by-product of new or more intense exercise.

41. T or F   Plyometric exercises are functionally appropriate exercises to use for all orthopedic patients.

42. T or F   Plyometrics are most often used to develop strength.

43. T or F   Plyometrics is a "system" of exercises that utilizes the myotatic stretch reflex and the neurophysiologic responses from the Golgi tendon organs (GTOs) and muscle spindles to create high-speed reaction forces and power.

44. T or F   Closed kinetic chain exercises must always be deferred until the final phase of recovery.

45. T or F   The human body functions as a combination of both open and closed kinetic chain activities.

46. T or F   High intensity strength training for the elderly is not safe nor effective and does not lead to improved function.

47. T or F   Studies demonstrate that muscle size (hypertrophy), strength (force-generation), and function (gait and balance) can be improved in the elderly with appropriately applied high intensity resistance exercise.

ESSAY QUESTIONS

Answer on a separate sheet of paper.

48. Name the noncontractile and contractile elements of muscle tissue.
49. Describe and contrast muscle fiber types.
50. Define types of muscle contraction.
51. Give examples of concentric and eccentric contractions.
52. Give two definitions of strength.
53. Define and clarify terms used to describe muscular performance.
54. List methods used to measure strength.
55. Compare muscle contraction types in relation to tension produced and energy liberated.
56. Discuss muscle response to exercise.
57. Identify clinical features of delayed onset muscle soreness (DOMS).
58. Discuss velocity spectrum training related to isokinetic exercise.
59. List three clinically relevant exercise programs used to enhance strength.

60. Discuss plyometrics.
61. Explain open and closed kinetic chain exercise.
62. Identify goals and applications of strength training programs for the elderly.

CRITICAL THINKING APPLICATION

In small groups, discuss and develop specific sequential sets of exercises and identify types of muscle contractions that will enhance quadriceps strength and power following a rectus femoris muscle strain. Which muscle contraction type would you recommend initially? Why? Which types of exercises would you encourage to stimulate type I muscle fiber? Which exercises would you encourage to stimulate type II muscle fiber?

Develop a continuum of exercises that appropriately addresses isometrics, concentric and eccentric contractions, and isokinetics. Give three clinically relevant examples of each contraction type and explain when and why you would use each. What is an anticipated by-product of your exercise continuum as you progress your patient from one contraction type to another? To prevent or minimize patellofemoral compressive loads during quad strengthening activities, what modifications, if any, would you recommend? Describe the appropriate application of closed kinetic chain exercises and plyometrics following recovery from a rectus femoris muscle strain.

Endurance

MULTIPLE CHOICE

1. Oxidative phosphorylation is capable of producing how many more times the amount of ATP than the anaerobic ATP-PC energy system?
   A. Five
   B. Ten
   C. Forty
   D. Nineteen
   E. Fifteen

2. The measurement of the efficiency of the aerobic system is called:
   A. Aerobic efficiency
   B. Vital capacity
   C. Maximum oxygen uptake (VO$_2$ max)
   D. Cardiovascular fitness

3. The capacity of an aerobic system to perform work is called:
   A. Aerobic capacity
   B. Cardiovascular fitness
   C. Cardiovascular endurance
   D. Cardiorespiratory fitness
   E. All of the above

4. Which of the following describes the changes that occur as a result of long-term aerobic exercise training? (circle any that apply)
   A. Increase in myosin ATPase
   B. Increase in mitochondria
   C. Selective hypertrophy of type II muscle fibers
   D. Blood volume and hemoglobin increased
   E. Atrophy of red muscle fiber

5. Which of the following describes the AAMHR?
   A. 120 − age = MHR
   B. 220 − age = MHR
   C. 220 + age = MHR
   D. 150 + age = MHR

6. The ACSM recommends the following intensity level for aerobic exercise in healthy adults:
   A. 50% to 80% of MHR
   B. 60% to 75% of MHR
   C. 60% to 90% of MHR
   D. 75% to 100% of MHR

7. The Borg scale is used to describe:
   A. Perceived exertion
   B. Actual, objective aerobic stress
   C. Exercise intensity
   D. None of the above

8. To elicit aerobic fitness a person must train:
   A. 2 to 3 days per week
   B. 1 to 3 days per week

C. 3 to 5 days per week

D. 2 to 4 days per week

9. To affect physiologic aerobic adaptations, the duration of exercise must be:

A. 5 to 10 minutes

B. 20 to 60 minutes

C. 15 to 20 minutes

D. 10 to 20 minutes

10. Aerobic exercise can be divided into two categories:

A. Rapid and slow

B. Long duration and short duration

C. Continuous and discontinuous

D. Intense and brief

11. If a patient is recovering from a lower extremity injury (with a cast), which of the following aerobic exercises can be safely employed? (circle any that apply)

A. Underwater treadmill

B. Single leg stationary cycle ergometer

C. Stair stepper

D. UBE

E. Slide board

12. For patients recovering from an injury to one upper extremity, which of the following aerobic exercise tools would be most appropriate? (circle any that apply)

A. One arm UBE

B. Stationary cycle

C. Treadmill

D. Upper extremity slideboard

E. Swimming

13. Aerobic conditioning is an important factor when recovering from injury or surgery of the lumbar spine. Which of the following may be most appropriate in this type of recovery? (circle any that apply)

A. Saddle seat stationary cycle ergometer

B. Recumbent seat ergometer

C. Treadmill

D. Underwater treadmill

E. Long distance running

TRUE/FALSE

14. T or F   Aerobic exercise is ill-advised for patients recovering from orthopedic injury or surgery.

ESSAY QUESTIONS

Answer on a separate sheet of paper.

15. Define VO_2 max.

16. List adaptive physiologic changes related to aerobic exercise.

17. Describe the age-adjusted maximum heart rate (AAMHR).

18. Discuss several guidelines for the development of aerobic fitness related to frequency, intensity, duration, and mode of activity.

19. Outline methods of aerobic training.

20. Identify orthopedic considerations during aerobic exercise.

21. Discuss two hypotheses that attempt to clarify peripheral neuromuscular fatigue as a result of prolonged or strenuous muscle activity.

22. Compare endurance training alone with the effects of a combined program of aerobic training and strength training.

CRITICAL THINKING APPLICATION

Describe various activities you would recommend to stimulate cardiovascular fitness for a patient recovering from a low back injury. Design an aerobic fitness program using three different modes of training that would be appropriate for this patient. Which methods would you use to prescribe and measure aerobic exercise? How would you determine the intensity and subsequent progression of the aerobic activities? Describe the frequency, intensity, and duration of cardiovascular exercise you would recommend in this case. How do progressive increases in the intensity of aerobic conditioning affect cardiovascular risk, orthopedic injury, and general exercise compliance? In prescribing aerobic conditioning programs, name 10 adaptive physiologic changes you would hope to affect.

By contrast, list three modes of cardiovascular fitness training for a patient with a knee joint replacement. What considerations are there when identifying the most appropriate mode of training for patients with various orthopedic conditions or limitations?

Rarely are strength and cardiovascular fitness prescribed independently of one another. Discuss the concept of specificity and the SAID principle and how they relate to the development of strength and aerobic fitness.

Balance and Coordination

Balance
Coordination
Kinesthesia
Proprioception
Joint displacement
Velocity and amplitude of joint motion
Pressure
Stretch and pain
Mechanoreceptor system
Ruffini mechanoreceptors
Pacinian mechanoreceptors
Free nerve endings
Afferent neural input
Minitrampoline
Biomechanical ankle platform system (BAPS)
Wobble board
Kinesthetic ability training device (KAT)
Physioball

MULTIPLE CHOICE

1. Proprioception and the mechanoreceptor system provide information concerning:
   A. Joint displacement
   B. Joint position, direction, and speed
   C. Pressure and stretch
   D. Pain
   E. All of the above
2. Pacinian mechanoreceptors are involved with:
   A. Pain detection
   B. Muscle tension
   C. Ligament tension and velocity of motion
   D. Vestibular input
   E. All of the above
3. Free nerve endings are type IV mechanoreceptors and are involved with:

A. Pain and inflammation
B. Posture
C. Muscle stretch
D. Ligament tension
E. None of the above

4. Type I mechanoreceptors are called Ruffini mechanoreceptors and are responsible for:
   A. High–speed position sense
   B. Muscle tension
   C. Static joint position
   D. Direction of joint motion
   E. None of the above
5. A critical safety component to all balance and proprioception activities is the patient's ability to demonstrate:
   A. Increased ROM
   B. Improved strength
   C. Protective reactions
   D. Faster gait
   E. All of the above
6. A challenging dynamic balance test and activity requires the patient to:
   A. Maintain balance with eyes closed while standing
   B. Ambulate and negotiate obstacles
   C. Maintain balance while seated, performing trunk rotation
   D. Maintain balance while seated, performing marching
7. Which of the following factors contributes to balance dysfunction?
   A. Perception
   B. Weakness
   C. Range of motion
   D. Coordination
   E. All of the above
8. Which of the following devices represents challenging tasks to improve balance and proprioception?
   A. KAT
   B. BAPS

C. Minitrampoline
D. Wobble board
E. All of the above

9. Which of the following exercises can be used for closed chain-proprioception activities following upper extremity injuries? (circle any that apply)
A. Push-ups
B. Minitrampoline
C. Physioball, or plyoball
D. Bicep curls
E. Pendulum exercises

SHORT ANSWER

10. Name two ways to increase the intensity of the double–leg stance test (DLST).
11. Studies have demonstrated that many falls occur in the elderly during walking, ascending and descending stairs, and during turns. Which activity and/or test would be most appropriate for developing single–leg stance equilibrium?
12. Organize the following balance and proprioception activities from the simplest (1) to the most challenging (5).
_____ Double-leg standing—eyes closed
_____ Standing—weight shifting
_____ Single-leg standing—eyes closed
_____ Sitting balance—eyes open
_____ Single-leg standing—eyes closed with manual resistance
13. List three plyoball exercises that can be used to increase dynamic trunk balance, proprioception, and strength.

TRUE/FALSE

14. T or F   The joint mechanoreceptor system (afferent neural input system) is important in regulating changes related to joint movement and body position.
15. T or F   SLST and DLST are examples of balance tests and are never used as treatment activities.
16. T or F   High–density foam padding is used for patients to stand and walk on during the final phase of balance training.
17. T or F   A high degree of balance is required to maintain equilibrium while standing and walking on low density foam.
18. T or F   The reach test shows the patient's ability to reach and challenge the limits or borders of the base of support.

19. T or F   Injury, surgery, immobilization, and non–weight bearing convalescence have a profoundly negative effect on the afferent neural input system.
20. T or F   Rehabilitation programs that do not address balance, coordination, and proprioception can result in poor restoration of function and increases the risk of reinjury.
21. T or F   Postoperative shoulder patients do not require proprioception exercises because the shoulder is a non–weight bearing structure.

ESSAY QUESTIONS

Answer on a separate sheet of paper.
22. Define and contrast balance and coordination.
23. Discuss the mechanoreceptor system and define four mechanoreceptors.
24. List static and dynamic balance and coordination tests and activities.
25. Define proprioception and kinesthetic awareness.
26. Discuss several factors that contribute to balance dysfunction.
27. Identify functional closed kinetic chain proprioceptive exercises.
28. Discuss the rationale for proprioceptive training for the upper extremity.

CRITICAL THINKING APPLICATION

To test and apply the principles of progressive balance tasks as described in Chapter 5 of the textbook, perform the following activity:

Stand on one leg with your eyes open. Now close your eyes.

What effect does visual input have on static balance? How does the mechanoreceptor system play a role in static and dynamic balance? What would happen to a patient's balance and proprioception following major ligament reconstruction of the knee? Outline and describe a specific sequence of progressively challenging and demanding balance and proprioception activities that would stimulate the afferent neural input system following knee ligament reconstructive surgery. Discuss how range of motion, weakness, and sensory input all contribute to balance dysfunction.

Describe the goals of closed chain-proprioception activities following injury or surgery to the upper extremity. Analyze why proprioception activities are encouraged for non–weight bearing structures such as the shoulder, elbow, and wrist. Develop a progressive series of proprioception activities that would follow glenohumeral dislocation.

II

Review of Tissue Healing

C H A P T E R

6

Ligament Healing

MULTIPLE CHOICE

1. Following injury, which type of collagen is predominantly produced?
   A. Type I
   B. Type III
   C. Type II
   D. Type IV

2. Long-term immobilization allows type III collagen to be:
   A. Arranged randomly
   B. Produced quickly
   C. Highly organized
   D. Quite strong

3. Active stress, muscular contractions, and joint motion allow collagen to be:
   A. Organized
   B. Stronger
   C. Functional
   D. All of the above

4. A sprain involves:
   A. Muscle
   B. Tendon
   C. Cartilage
   D. Ligament
   E. All of the above

5. Partial tearing of ligament fibers with resultant moderate joint laxity defines a:

   A. Grade II sprain
   B. Grade I sprain
   C. Grade III sprain
   D. None of the above

6. Which of the following are the most common of all ligament sprain classifications?
   A. Grades II and III
   B. Grades I and II
   C. Grades I and III
   D. Grades I, II, and III equally

7. Untreated ligament tears are:
   A. Composed primarily of type III collagen
   B. Biochemically inferior to ligaments treated with mobilization
   C. Generally not healed even 40 weeks after injury
   D. All of the above

8. Stress deprivation to ligaments leads to: (circle any that apply)
   A. Improved healing
   B. Secure collagen formation
   C. Ligament atrophy
   D. Reduced ligament strength
   E. Hypertrophy of ligament tissue

9. Some degree of immobilization is generally required to promote ligament healing. However, which of the following methods would also be appropriate for ligament healing without promoting the negative effects of immobilization? (circle any that apply)
   A. Limited range of motion braces
   B. Gentle, protected motion
   C. Rigid, secure plaster casting for 6 to 8 weeks
   D. Full ROM closed kinetic chain resistance exercise

10. Motion, stress, and general physical activity for healing ligaments (within defined and prescribed limits that do not adversely affect healing) result in: (circle any that apply)
    A. Reduced ligament weight
    B. Increased tensile strength of the ligament
    C. Arthrofibrosis

D. Hypertrophy
E. Random collagen alignment

11. Which type of exercise has been shown to be more effective in producing larger diameter collagen in ligaments?
A. Isometric
B. Concentric
C. Endurance type exercises
D. Eccentric

12. Studies show that joints that are moved passively (within carefully defined limits of motion that do not adversely affect healing) have:
A. More adhesions
B. More bleeding
C. Well-organized, longitudinally oriented collagen without adhesions
D. Reduced ligament strength
E. None of the above

13. CPM (continuous passive motion) is used for which of the following conditions?
A. ACL reconstructions
B. Total knee arthroplasty
C. Knee, elbow, and ankle fractures
D. Following long-term immobilization
E. All of the above

14. The concept of early protected motion following immobilization or surgery is to enhance and facilitate: (circle any that apply)
A. Muscular strength
B. Reduced bloody effusion within the joint
C. Increase connective tissue strength
D. Inhibit adhesions
E. Organized collagen alignment

SHORT ANSWER

15. Name the three phases of tissue healing.
16. Name the five cardinal signs of inflammation.
17. Organization and production of collagen occur during which phase of healing?
18. In order for torn ligaments to heal properly, the torn ends must be in _____ to one another. To orient collagen fibers and promote a "functional" scar, _____ must be applied. In addition, following injury or surgery to a ligament, protection against _____ must be strictly enforced.
19. Discuss the rationale for continuing or discontinuing external support as it relates to the healing constraints of ligament tissue following 2 weeks of progressive rehabilitation for a ligament sprain of the ankle.

TRUE/FALSE

20. T or F   Ligaments heal through a process of tissue regeneration.
21. T or F   Strict, long-term, rigid cast immobilization is necessary to allow for proper ligament healing.
22. T or F   The specific type and duration of exercise used during rehabilitation is not related to ligament and ligament-bone complex strength.
23. T or F   The long-term detrimental effects of immobilization on ligament and ligament-bone complex are not reversible.
24. T or F   Pain is an excellent guide to judge the degree of healing a ligament has achieved.
25. T or F   Ligaments may take a year or more to remodel and mature after surgery or injury.

ESSAY QUESTIONS

Answer on a separate sheet of paper.
26. Define and discuss the inflammatory response to injury.
27. Describe the phases of healing and the sequence of events characteristic to each phase of healing.
28. Identify the five cardinal signs of inflammation.
29. Describe the effects of immobilization on ligaments.
30. Discuss the effects of stress and exercise on ligaments.
31. Identify and discuss practical clinical applications of stress deprivation and protected motion during phases of ligament healing.

CRITICAL THINKING APPLICATION

Develop your own "case study" concerning a patient who has a grade II MCL sprain of the knee. Based on your knowledge of the mechanisms of ligament healing, recommend the application of rehabilitation procedures (immobilization, protected motion, bracing, resistance exercise, aerobic conditioning, proprioception, balance training, etc.) in an orderly sequence consistent with the inflammatory response, repair phase, and remodeling phase of tissue healing. In doing so, ask these questions: How do stress and stress deprivation affect collagen? How long should external bracing or support be considered and why? How does immobilization affect ligament tissue? What does protected motion refer to?

CHAPTER 7

Bone Healing

KEY TERMS

Salter-Harris fractures
Pathologic fractures
Osteoporosis
Osteomalacia
Spongy bone
Compact bone
Cancellous bone
Cortical bone
Osteoblasts
Osteocytes
Osteoclasts
Remodeling
Wolff's law
Piezoelectric effect
Bone callus
Immobilization
Delayed union
Nonunion
Malunion
External fixation devices
Internal fixation devices
Open reduction with internal fixation (ORIF)

MULTIPLE CHOICE

1. Which of the following describe(s) basic objectives in fracture management and healing? (circle any that apply)
   A. Muscular hypertrophy
   B. Approximate bone fragments
   C. Maintain alignment of fracture fragments
   D. Preserve and restore function
   E. Enhance aerobic metabolism

2. The adult skeleton is composed of what percent of compact, cortical bone?
   A. 10%
   B. 30%
   C. 80%
   D. 55%

3. Cells that help synthesize bone are called:
   A. Osteones
   B. Osteoclasts
   C. Osteocytes
   D. Osteoblasts

4. Immobilization and reduced physiological stress have what affect on healing bone tissue?
   A. Increased callus formation
   B. Stronger bone
   C. Increased osteoblast activity
   D. Decreased osteoblasts and rapid osteoclast activity

5. Normal bone growth, remodeling, and repair are influenced by:
   A. Motion
   B. Stress (Wolff's law)
   C. Muscular contractions
   D. Piezoelectric effect
   E. All of the above

6. Three complications that can arise from the process of bone healing are: (circle any that apply)
   A. Decreased cardiorespiratory function
   B. Delayed union
   C. Nonunion
   D. Malunion
   E. Hard callus formation

7. Which of the following are descriptive classifications of fractures? (circle any that apply)
   A. Injury site
   B. Force of injury
   C. Configuration of injury

D. Relationship of fracture fragments to the environment

E. Resultant functional deficits

8. Which of the following are classifications of pediatric fractures?
   A. Smith-Harris
   B. Salter-James
   C. Salter-Harris
   D. Harris-Jones

9. Which is the most common cause of pathologic fractures?
   A. Tumors
   B. Stress fractures
   C. Metastatic bone disease
   D. Osteoporosis

10. Osteoporosis is characterized by: (circle any that apply)
    A. Decreased quality of bone
    B. Increased quantity of bone
    C. Osteoclast activity greater than osteoblast activity
    D. Decreased quantity of bone
    E. Increased tensile strength of bone

11. The most common pathologic fracture related to osteoporosis is:
    A. Humeral neck fractures
    B. Stress fractures
    C. Vertebral body compression fractures
    D. Colles' fractures

12. Which of the following are methods of external fixation of fractures? (circle any that apply)
    A. Traction
    B. Pins
    C. Screws
    D. Cast-braces
    E. Harrington rods

13. The method of open reduction and internal fixation of fractures is known as what type of procedure? (circle any that apply)
    A. ORIF
    B. Reduction with fixation
    C. A surgical procedure to internally stabilize a fracture
    D. A surgical procedure used only to stabilize open or compound fractures

14. Which of the following exercises are commonly used for the immobilized area during recovery from fractures?
    A. High-speed isokinetics
    B. Eccentrics
    C. Isometrics
    D. Concentrics

15. When cast-braces are used (protected limited range), occasionally the physician and physical therapist will prescribe what type of muscular activity during the early recovery phase of rehabilitation? (circle any that apply)
    A. Isometrics
    B. Active range of motion
    C. Isokinetics
    D. Plyometrics
    E. Closed kinetic chain eccentric loading

16. What adjunctive technique is occasionally used to encourage, stimulate, and enhance muscular contractions during periods of cast immobilization for the treatment of fractures?
    A. Ultrasound
    B. Phonophoresis
    D. TENS
    E. Electrical muscle stimulation (EMS)

17. Exercise is a significant feature of recovery following fractures. Appropriately applied muscular contractions provide which of the following during recovery from fractures?
    A. Improved circulation
    B. Fragment approximation
    C. Promote motion to nonimmobilization parts
    D. Stimulate the piezoelectric effect
    E. All of the above

18. Which of the following are general goals of recovery during the immobilization of fractures?
    A. Improve patient fitness
    B. Minimize muscular atrophy
    C. Protect healing structures
    D. Teach safe and effective gait and transfers
    E. All of the above

SHORT ANSWER

19. Name the two general methods used to immobilize fractures.

20. When treating a patient with an ORIF procedure in which a screw was used to stabilize a fracture, the PTA must be cautious of hardware loosening and "backing out." List three clinical signs of hardware loosening.

TRUE/FALSE

21. T or F   Compact bone heals faster than cancellous bone.

22. T or F   A reduced rate of bone healing (delayed union) can happen when physical therapy

interventions are applied too soon or too vigorously.

23. T or F   When treating patients recovering from fractures, it is necessary to actively exercise all nonimmobilized joints.

ESSAY QUESTIONS

Answer on a separate sheet of paper.

24. Identify and describe the phases of bone healing.
25. Discuss the objectives that serve as the foundation of fracture management and bone healing.
26. Define osteoblasts, osteoclasts, and osteocytes.
27. Define and discuss Wolff's law.
28. Discuss stress deprivation, immobilization, and normal physiologic stress as they apply to fracture healing.
29. Define three complications of bone healing.
30. Outline and describe six areas of descriptive organization of classifying fractures.
31. Describe the five types of pediatric fractures defined by Salter-Harris.
32. Define pathologic fractures and list four types.
33. Discuss how osteoporosis affects fractures.
34. Define osteomalacia.

35. List common methods of fracture fixation, fixation devices, and fracture classifications.
36. Discuss clinical applications of rehabilitation techniques used during bone healing.

CRITICAL THINKING APPLICATION

Develop your own "case study" concerning a patient with a distal tibia fracture. Based on your knowledge of the mechanisms of bone healing, recommend the application of specific rehabilitation procedures (immobilization, protected motion, weight bearing, resistance exercise, aerobic conditioning, proprioception and balance training, etc.) that are consistent with the phases of bone healing and remodeling.

Identify the influence of Wolff's law on bone remodeling. In developing your rehabilitation program, consider the effects of immobilization of bone and describe clinically significant complications that could occur following fractures. Identify when an ORIF procedure is generally indicated for fracture stabilization. During each phase of recovery in your case study, address the following issues: the overall fitness of the patient, minimization of muscle atrophy, improvement of muscular strength, and protection of the healing structures.

Cartilage Healing

Hyaline cartilage
Osteoarthritis
Chondrocytes
Subchondral bone
Inflammatory response
Continuous passive motion (CPM)
Meniscus injury and repair
Fibroelastic cartilage
Meniscectomy
Zone I
Red-on-red
Zone II
Red-on-white
Zone III
White-on-white
"Vascular access channel"

MULTIPLE CHOICE

1. What percent of articular cartilage is water?
   A. 10% to 20%
   B. 65% to 80%
   C. 35% to 50%
   D. 15% to 40%
2. Which of the following characterizes articular cartilage?
   A. Frictionless
   B. 2 to 4 mm thick (generally)
   C. Quite durable—resistant to wear
   D. Able to dissipate compressive loads many times greater than body weight
   E. All of the above

3. Which of the following describe(s) how articular cartilage can become damaged? (circle any that apply)
   A. Joint instability
   B. Immobilization
   C. Fever
   D. Repetitive overload
   E. Non-weight bearing and reduced physiologic loading
4. Which of the following describe(s) how joint immobilization affects articular cartilage? (circle any that apply)
   A. Increased articular wear
   B. Increased friction abrasion
   C. Loss of proteoglyca
   D. Reduced mechanical loading leading to degeneration
   E. Improved healing of superficial wounds
5. Which of the following characterize(s) how significant articular cartilage lesions heal? (circle any that apply)
   A. Reduced blood supply to deep lesion
   B. Reduced inflammatory response
   C. Increased vascular supply to lesion
   D. Chondrocytes communicate with the wound
   E. Reduced chondrocytes in deep wounds
6. Femoral and retropatellar arthroscopic abrasion is designed to: (circle any that apply)
   A. Promote articular cartilage repair with deep-significant wounds
   B. Smooth the articular surface
   C. Stimulate the inflammatory process
   D. Elicit repair via subchondral bone bleeding
   E. Improve patellofemoral joint stability

7. Which of the following describes the functions of the meniscus?
   A. Dissipation of compressive loads
   B. Joint lubrication
   C. Load bearing
   D. Joint stability
   E. All of the above
8. Degenerative tears of the meniscus occurs typically to people:
   A. Younger than 30 years old
   B. Older than 40 years old
   C. Older than 30 years old, but younger than 40 years old
   D. Between 70 and 80 years old
9. Which of the following describes the mechanism of injury of an intraarticular fibrocartilage tear?
   A. Twisting
   B. Torque
   C. Deceleration
   D. Compression
   E. All of the above
10. What percentage of the periphery is vascular in the medial and lateral meniscus?
   A. 5% to 10%
   B. 40% to 50%
   C. 10% to 30%
   D. 20% to 40%
11. What percentage of meniscal tears occurs in the vascular border of the meniscus?
   A. 5%
   B. 40%
   C. 15% to 20%
   D. 10%
12. If an injury occurs to an area of the meniscus where the tear is vascular on both sides, it is called: (circle any that apply)
   A. Reparable
   B. Red on white
   C. Red on red
   D. Non-reparable
   E. Zone III
13. Which zones of injury are considered reparable? (circle any that apply)
   A. Red-on-white
   B. White-on-white
   C. Red-on-red
   D. Zone II
   E. Zone I
14. Identify the characteristics of rehabilitation following an isolated meniscal repair as compared with total or sub-total meniscectomy: (circle any that apply)

A. Long-term goals are basically the same
B. Weight bearing and full range of motion should be deferred until secure healing has occurred
C. Closed chain exercises begin two weeks following repair
D. Full weight bearing is allowed as soon as pain allows
E. Full knee flexion allowed one week post-op

SHORT ANSWER

15. Name the three classic surgical procedures used to correct tears of the meniscus.
16. The meniscus of the knee can be injured in two distinct ways. Name the two classifications of meniscal injuries.

TRUE/FALSE

17. T or F   If an injury were to occur to the central nonvascular portion of the meniscus, spontaneous intrinsic repair is not possible.
18. T or F   Normal joint motion and compressive loads are necessary for hyaline (articular) cartilage to remain viable.
19. T or F   The deeper and more extensive the damage to articular cartilage, the less "healing" occurs.
20. T or F   Superficial articular cartilage lesions heal much quicker and to a greater degree than significant wounds.
21. T or F   CPM is used to help stimulate cartilage nutrition in partial-thickness articular cartilage lesions.
22. T or F   The meniscus of the knee serves as a primary joint restraint.
23. T or F   The central portion of the medial and lateral meniscus are essentially avascular.

ESSAY QUESTIONS

Answer on a separate sheet of paper.
24. Discuss the composition and function of articular cartilage.
25. Identify common causes of injury to articular cartilage.
26. Describe the sequence of healing and the extent of intrinsic repair of articular cartilage.
27. Define invasive and noninvasive techniques of stimulating articular cartilage repair.
28. Define and describe the composition and function of the meniscus.

29. Identify and discuss common mechanisms of injury to the meniscus.
30. Describe the mechanisms of intrinsic healing of the meniscus.
31. List common rehabilitation techniques used in the treatment of the injured meniscus.

CRITICAL THINKING APPLICATION

Develop your own "case study" concerning a patient with superficial articular cartilage degeneration of the patellofemoral joint. Based on your knowledge of the mechanisms of articular cartilage healing, recommend the application of rehabilitation techniques (immobilization, protected motion, CPM, range of motion, resistance exercise, closed kinetic chain exercises, aerobic conditioning, proprioception and balance training, etc.) that are consistent with the stages of articular cartilage repair. Make specific reference to modification in exercise and functional activities based on your knowledge of patellofemoral compressive forces during the performance of various open and closed chain activities. In developing your program, ask these questions: How do more significant articular cartilage defects heal in comparison to superficial wounds? Is physiologic motion necessary for the nutrition of articular cartilage?

List invasive surgical techniques used to stimulate subchondral bone bleeding in cases of femoral and patellar articular cartilage disease.

In terms of a meniscal injury, develop a list of reasons related to motion, weight bearing and closed chain functional activities that contrast the rationale for alteration in rehabilitation between meniscal repairs and subtotal meniscectomy.

CHAPTER 9

Muscle and Tendon Healing

KEY TERMS

Sprain
Strain
Microtrauma
Overuse
Indirect muscle injury
Direct muscle injury
Contusion
Incomplete muscle tears
Complete muscle tears
Immobilization
Atrophy
Tendinitis
Tenocytes
Protected motion

MULTIPLE CHOICE

1. Which of the following is most susceptible to indirect, incomplete muscle strains?
   A. Muscle belly
   B. Biceps
   C. Quadriceps
   D. Musculotendinous junction
2. Which type of muscle contraction is a frequent cause of indirect muscle strain? (circle any that apply)
   A. Isometric
   B. Isokinetic
   C. Concentric
   D. Eccentric
   E. Isotonic
3. The most profound change in human skeletal muscle during immobilization is atrophy. The degree of muscle atrophy depends on:

A. The significance of the injury
B. The type of surgical procedure
C. The duration of immobilization and the position or stretch imposed on the limb during immobilization
D. The amount of bleeding

4. Which type of muscle fiber atrophies to a great degree when muscle is immobilized in a shortened position?
   A. Type I—slow twitch
   B. Type II—fast twitch
   C. Fast twitch—A
   D. Fast twitch—AB
   E. Fast twitch—B
5. An increase in sarcomeres up to 20% as well as protein synthesis is seen when muscle is:
   A. Immobilized for 6 weeks or longer
   B. Immobilized in a lengthened position
   C. Immobilized in a shortened position
   D. Not severely damaged
6. The healing response of muscle is:
   A. The same as bone
   B. Less than ligaments
   C. Similar to cartilage
   D. Greater than bone, ligament, or cartilage
7. The use of electrically evoked muscle stimulation in conjunction with isometric muscle contractions during periods of immobilization may: (circle any that apply)
   A. Retard disuse atrophy
   B. Minimize strength loss
   C. Reduce the loss of succinic dehydrogenase
   D. Enhance cardiovascular fitness
   E. Greatly enhance eccentric strength
8. When a severe, deep muscle contusion occurs, it is wise to avoid heat, early progressive motion, or massage because:

A. These treatments are too painful

B. These treatments are ineffective for pain and swelling relief

C. These treatments may promote myositis ossificans (MOT)

D. Motion can effectively eliminate a hematoma by itself

9. Tendons heal by way of three organized stages of inflammation, repair, and remodeling. However, tendons have the capacity to heal:

A. By inflammatory response only

B. By intrinsic repair only

C. By extrinsic repair only

D. By both intrinsic and extrinsic repair

10. A tendon generally receives its blood supply from: (circle any that apply)

A. The muscle belly

B. Bone

C. Synovium

D. Musculotendinous junction

E. Articular surfaces

11. Which of the following describes the effects of early, limited, and protective motion during tendon healing?

A. Decreased tendon strength

B. Reduced bone strength

C. Less adhesion formation

D. Increased gap formation

12. Which of the following describes a common course of rehabilitation for cases of tendonitis?

A. Surgery, immobilization-rehab

B. RICE, protection, progressive exercise

C. Full ROM, active exercise

D. Rigid immobilization

13. Tendon injuries that require surgical repair are best treated with:

A. Nonrestrictive full-range-of-motion exercises after immobilization

B. Temporary rigid immobilization followed by closed chain resistance exercise

C. Limited immobilization; gentle-protected range of motion; and appropriate exercise

D. Rigid, long-term immobilization, non–weight bearing, followed by unlimited exercise

SHORT ANSWER

14. A muscle injury that occurs as a result of sudden stretch (concentric or eccentric muscle contraction) is referred to as _____ .

15. A muscle injury that occurs as a result of a contusion, laceration, or surgical incision is called _____ .

TRUE/FALSE

16. T or F   Generally, muscle tissue heals by way of intense, acute inflammatory response.

17. T or F   Indirect, incomplete muscle strains are more common than complete muscle strains.

18. T or F   If a muscle is immobilized in a shortened position, it will atrophy more than if the muscle were placed in a lengthened or stretched position.

19. T or F   Concentric and eccentric muscle contractions can be used in selected cases with range-limiting hinged cast-braces.

20. T or F   Controlled motion, limited stress, and appropriately applied exercise are necessary adjuncts during periods of tendon healing.

21. T or F   Tendinitis is best treated with surgical excision and periods of immobilization.

ESSAY QUESTIONS

Answer on a separate sheet of paper.

22. Define and contrast the terms *sprain* and *strain*.

23. Discuss direct and indirect muscle injuries.

24. Define and describe complete and incomplete muscle injuries.

25. Identify and describe the sequence of muscle injury repair.

26. List the effects of immobilization of muscle tissue.

27. Describe clinically relevant rehabilitation techniques used during periods of muscle injury, repair, and immobilization.

28. Define and describe the organized stages of tendon healing.

29. Contrast the intrinsic and extrinsic capacity of tendon tissue to heal.

30. Outline and describe the effects of motion and immobilization on tendons.

31. Discuss the clinical applications of rehabilitation techniques during tendon healing.

CRITICAL THINKING APPLICATION

Based on your understanding of the mechanisms of muscle injury and repair, develop a list of rehabilitation techniques you would recommend following immobilization, indirect muscle strain, and direct muscle injury. Organize and construct a working rehabilitation plan that focuses attention on the restoration of motion, soft tissue extensibility, strength, power, neuromuscular endurance, cardiovascular fitness, proprioception and balance, and functional closed kinetic chain exercises.

Be certain to categorize your therapeutic interventions so that they are consistent with the stages of muscle tissue healing and time constraints. What adjunctive techniques would you recommend to stimulate muscle reeducation? Which thermal agents would you encourage during each phase of muscle healing? Are there any contraindications for employing massage, heat, and passive motion following a muscle injury? Explain. Describe in detail the specific application of isometric, concentric, and eccentric muscle contractions during each phase of intrinsic muscle repair.

Describe the clinical rationale for use of early protected motion versus immobilization following tendon injury or surgical repair.

Gait and Joint Mobilization

Fundamentals of Gait

KEY TERMS

Gait
Base of support
Center of gravity
Step length
Cadence
Stride length
Stance phase
Swing phase
Double support
Single support
Pelvic "list"
Heel strike
Foot flat
Mid-stance
Heel-off
Toe-off
Acceleration
Mid-swing
Deceleration
Antalgic gait
Steppage gait
Trendelenburg gait
Abductor "lurch"
Calcaneal gait
Four-point gait pattern
Three-point gait pattern
Two-point gait pattern
Non-weight-bearing (NWB)
Partial weight bearing (PWB)
Touch-down weight bearing (TDWB)
Toe-touch weight bearing (TTWB)
Weight bearing as tolerated (WBAT)
Full-weight bearing (FWB)

MULTIPLE CHOICE

1. In terms of gait, a wider base of support provides:
   A. Greater endurance
   B. Less stability
   C. Reduced trunk motion
   D. Greater stability
2. An individual's center of gravity is:
   A. Unchanged during gait
   B. Approximately 5 cm anterior to the second sacral vertebrae
   C. Unimportant and unrelated to stability
   D. Located in the upper lumbar vertebrae
3. The number of total steps per minute during gait is called:
   A. Stride length
   B. Cadence
   C. Gait cycle
   D. None of the above
4. Which of the following represents approximately 60% of the entire gait cycle?
   A. Stride length
   B. Stance phase
   C. Swing phase
   D. Double support
5. The swing phase of gait occupies what percentage of the gait cycle?
   A. 10%
   B. 20%
   C. 15%
   D. 40%
   E. 60%
6. The pelvis rotates within the frontal plane of the body during gait. This pelvic rotation is termed:

A. List
B. Pitch
C. Yaw
D. Pelvic deviation

7. The stance phase of gait has how many components?
A. 3
B. 4
C. 5
D. 6

8. The swing phase of gait has how many components?
A. 4
B. 2
C. 3
D. 5

9. During the stance phase of gait,_____ is the instant foot contact is made with the ground.
A. Foot-flat
B. Heel-off
C. Heel-strike
D. Mid-stance

10. During the stance phase of gait,_____ is the time when the entire foot is in contact with the ground.
A. Mid-stance
B. Foot-flat
C. Heel-off
D. Toe-off

11. What is the name of the period where the body is directly over the weight-bearing leg?
A. Toe-off
B. Heel-strike
C. Mid-stance
D. Heel-off

12. _____ is when weight is unloaded from the weight-bearing limb and transferred to the opposite limb.
A. Toe-off
B. Heel-off
C. Mid-stance
D. Heel-strike

13. A painful gait pattern is referred to as:
A. A steppage gait
B. An antalgic gait
C. An abductor lurch
D. None of the above

14. A rapid swing phase of the uninvolved limb, with a reduction of the stance phase of the involved limb is characteristic of which type of gait?
A. Antalgic gait
B. Steppage gait

C. Trendelenburg gait
D. Abductor lurch

15. Weakness of the tibialis anterior, and excessive hip flexion and knee flexion during swing-through, are characteristic deviations to prevent toe drag. What is this gait pattern called?
A. Trendelenburg gait
B. Antalgic gait
C. Steppage gait
D. None of the above

16. Weakness of the gluteus medius results in a(n):
A. Abductor lurch
B. Trendelenburg gait
C. Rapid swing through
D. Steppage gait
E. A and B

17. Circumduction of the hip during swing-through is characteristic of weakness to which muscle group?
A. Quadriceps
B. Hip flexors (psoas)
C. Gluteus medius
D. Hip abductors

18. Weakness of which muscle group will demonstrate knee hyperextension during the stance phase of the gait cycle?
A. Hamstrings
B. Hip flexors
C. Hip adductors
D. Quadriceps

19. Which of the following describes a four-point gait pattern, if the injured limb is the left leg?
A. Right crutch → left crutch → right foot → left foot
B. Left crutch → right foot → right crutch → left foot
C. Right crutch → left foot → left crutch → right foot
D. Left crutch → right crutch → left foot → right foot

20. TDWB is described as:
A. Minimal weight bearing (balance only)
B. Moderate weight bearing
C. 30% weight bearing
D. None of the above

21. WBAT is designed for patients who are limited by which factors?
A. Muscle strength
B. ORIF procedures
C. Non-surgical injuries
D. Pain

22. When instructing a patient to ascend stairs with bilateral axillary crutches, which of the following describes the most appropriate sequence?
A. Involved limb, then crutches
B. Crutches, then uninvolved limb

C. Uninvolved limb, then crutches

D. Crutches, then involved limb

23. When descending stairs using bilateral axillary crutches, which of the following describes the most appropriate sequence?

    A. Crutches first, then the uninjured limb

    B. Involved limb, then crutches

    C. Uninvolved limb, then crutches

    D. Crutches, then involved limb

24. When descending stairs, the physical therapist assistant should stand and provide support:

    A. To the uninvolved side of the patient

    B. To the involved side of the patient

    C. In front of the patient

    D. Behind the patient

25. When ascending stairs, the physical therapist assistant should stand and provide support:

    A. To the involved side

    B. To the uninvolved side

    C. Behind the patient

    D. In front of the patient

SHORT ANSWER

26. What is the term used to describe linear distance between right and left feet during gait?

27. Name the two phases of gait.

28. Name the components of the stance phase of gait.

29. Name the components of the swing phase of gait.

30. Name a primary action of the foot-flat period of the stance phase of gait.

31. A single crutch or cane should be used on which side of the injured limb?

TRUE/FALSE

32. T or F   During gait, an individual's center of gravity displaces both vertically and horizontally.

33. T or F   NWB status allows the patient to place minimal weight on the involved limb.

34. T or F   PWB status allows the patient to place a prescribed amount of resistance on the

involved limb. The amount of weight is determined by the physician and is carried out in physical therapy by grading the resistance by a percentage of the patient's weight (20%, 30%, 50%, etc.).

ESSAY QUESTIONS

Answer on a separate sheet of paper.

35. Define and describe basic components of the gait cycle.

36. Discuss the two phases of gait.

37. Identify and describe each component of the two phases of gait.

38. Define and describe common gait deviations.

39. Define and describe three appropriate gait patterns.

40. Outline and describe terms used to define weight-bearing status during gait.

41. Identify and discuss the appropriate use of assistive devices for ascending and descending stairs.

CRITICAL THINKING APPLICATION

You are treating a patient with right quadriceps atrophy and a 40% loss of knee extension strength. The physical therapist has asked you to initiate gait instruction using bilateral axillary crutches; a three-point gait pattern and the patient's weight-bearing status is as tolerated (WBAT).

During which phase of the gait cycle would you anticipate observable clinical manifestations of this patient's problem? What muscle contraction type is required of the quadriceps during heel strike? Which action of the knee does quadriceps strength control?

After a few weeks, this patient develops an additional gait deviation, and you notice the pelvis dropping toward the unaffected side during single limb support of the stance phase. Which muscle group(s) are affected, and what is the name of this gait pattern?

When instructing this patient to ascend and descend stairs, describe precisely the techniques you would instruct the patient to use if no handrails were available. Where would you position yourself during stair climbing and descent? Why?

Concepts of Joint Mobilization

KEY TERMS

Mobilization
Glide
Spin
Slide
Roll
Physiologic joint motion
Accessory joint motion
"Joint play"
Joint congruency
Close-packed
Loose-packed
Convex-concave rule
Velocity
Oscillation
Amplitude of movement
Traction
Piccolo traction
Bone to bone
Soft-tissue approximation
Hard or springy-tissue stretch
Muscle spasm
Springy block
Empty end-feel
Loose end-feel
Capsular end-feel
Capsular pattern
Noncapsular pattern

MULTIPLE CHOICE

1. Which of the following best describes physiological joint motions of the knee?
   A. Roll
   B. Spin
   C. Flexion-extension
   D. Glide

2. Which of the following best describes accessory movements? (circle any that apply)
   A. Flexion
   B. Extension
   C. Spin
   D. Glide
   E. Roll

3. How many grades of physiological and accessory joint motions has Maitland described?
   A. 3
   B. 5
   C. 6
   D. 8

4. Which of the following terms is(are) used to describe the degree of force and rate of motion used during the performance of joint mobilization? (circle any that apply)
   A. Strength
   B. Power
   C. Velocity and amplitude
   D. Oscillation
   E. Eccentrics

5. A large amplitude motion that occurs from the mid–range of motion to the end of the available range is a:
   A. Grade II mobilization
   B. Grade I mobilization
   C. Grade III mobilization
   D. Grade IV mobilization

6. A small oscillation or small amplitude joint motion that occurs only at the beginning of the available range of motion is a:
   A. Grade III mobilization
   B. Grade I mobilization

C. Grade II mobilization

D. Grade IV mobilization

7. A small oscillation or amplitude of motion that occurs at the end-range of available motion is a:

A. Grade IV mobilization

B. Grade III mobilization

C. Grade V mobilization

D. Grade II mobilization

8. A large amplitude of motion that occurs from the mid–range of motion to the end of the available range is considered:

A. Grade I

B. Grade III

C. Grade II

D. Grade V

E. Grade IV

9. In general terms, which grades of mobilization are used to treat painful joint motions?

A. Grades II and III

B. Grades I and III

C. Grades I and II

D. Grades II and IV

10. When performing passive range of motion to a joint, a sudden nonyielding, hard end-range feel is described as:

A. Myositis ossificans

B. Hard or springy tissue stretch

C. Bone to bone end-feel

D. Soft-tissue approximation

11. Terminal knee extension and wrist flexion describe the most common normal feel at the end range of joints. This is called:

A. Bone to bone

B. Springy tissue stretch

C. Soft-tissue approximation

D. Joint play

12. A characteristic end-range feel during knee flexion or elbow flexion at the end range of motion is called:

A. Soft-tissue approximation

B. Springy tissue-stretch

C. Joint play

D. Rising tension

13. An abnormal end-feel that is characterized by pain and a sudden halt of motion is called:

A. Capsular end-feel

B. Empty end-feel

C. Springy block

D. Muscle spasm

14. An abnormal end-feel, which is characterized by a lack of resistance at the end range of motion, signifying extreme joint laxity, is called:

A. Empty end-feel

B. Loose end-feel

C. Capsular end-feel

D. Springy block

15. An abnormal end-feel, which is characterized by limited motion, pain without muscle spasm, and without any mechanical block or restriction, is called:

A. Capsular end-feel

B. Elastic resistance

C. Empty end-feel

D. Springy block

16. A painful resistance at the end-range of motion accompanied by a soft sensation is called:

A. Elastic resistance

B. Springy block

C. Capsular end-feel

D. Empty end-feel

17. When elastic resistance is felt prior to the normal end range of motion, this is called:

A. Muscle spasm

B. Loose end-feel

C. Capsular end-feel

D. Springy block

18. All synovial joints under muscular control have unique, characteristic patterns of limitation. This is called:

A. Capsular pattern

B. Noncapsular pattern

C. Synergistic limitations

D. None of the above

19. When a lesion causes a restriction of motion that does not correspond to a characteristic, predetermined capsular pattern, this is called:

A. Joint laxity

B. Noncapsular pattern

C. Joint hypomobility

D. Nonspecific joint restriction

20. Which of the following are examples of possible causes of noncapsular pattern restrictions? (circle any that apply)

A. Ligament injury

B. Muscular weakness

C. Internal joint derangement

D. Extraarticular lesions

E. Vascular insufficiency

21. Which of the following is a relative contraindication for the application of joint mobilization?

A. Local bone disease

B. Active inflammatory arthritis

C. Osteoporosis

D. Malignancy

E. All of the above

22. Which of the following represent(s) absolute contraindications for the application of joint mobilization? (circle any that apply)
    A. Rheumatoid arthritis
    B. Infectious arthritis
    C. Joint hypermobility
    D. Central nervous system signs
    E. Malignancy of the area treated
23. Which of the following can be applied prior to the application of mobilization techniques to reduce tension and aid in relaxation of the patient?
    A. Hot packs
    B. Ultrasound
    C. Exercise
    D. TENS and EMS
    E. All of the above

SHORT ANSWER

24. When the concave surface is stationary and the convex surface is moving, the gliding movement in the joint occurs in a direction _____ to the bone movement.
25. When the convex surface is fixed, while the concave surface is mobile, the gliding motion occurs in the _____ direction as the bone movement.

TRUE/FALSE

26. T or F   When performing joint range of motion, the physical therapist assistant should encourage the patient to perform all accessory joint motions.
27. T or F   The "closed-packed" joint position is best used for determining joint stability.
28. T or F   The "loose-packed" position is best used for joint mobilization techniques.
29. T or F   Immediately following surgery, when pain may be significant, it is always appropriate to use grades I and II mobilization to help decrease pain.

ESSAY QUESTIONS

Answer on a separate sheet of paper.
30. Discuss the general and applied concepts of peripheral gait mobilization.
31. Define the terms and principles of peripheral joint mobilization.
32. Define and describe the convex-concave rule.
33. List and define the five grades of mobilization.
34. Identify and describe the terms of joint end-range feel.
35. Define and describe capsular and noncapsular patterns.
36. Identify common indications and contraindications for mobilization.
37. Discuss the clinical basis and applications of peripheral joint mobilization.
38. Identify and discuss the role of the PTA in assisting the physical therapist with the delivery of peripheral joint mobilization.

CRITICAL THINKING APPLICATION

You are asked by the physical therapist to prepare a patient for the application of peripheral joint mobilization techniques to the patient's left knee. Using a partner, perform this activity by demonstrating appropriate patient positioning, draping, and limb exposure. List adjunctive techniques that might be appropriate for patient relaxation, pain relief, compliance, and soft tissue extensibility. Outline and describe closed-packed and loose-packed positions in reference to this case.

Prior to the application of mobilization, the physical therapist instructed you to perform passive joint range of motion to this patient's knee. Define and describe the components of physiological movement and contrast these with accessory joint movements. Give examples of each. Describe the convex-concave rule. During the application of passive range of motion, you note a yielding compression during knee flexion. Define and describe this end-feel and give examples of two other distinct nonpathologic end-range feels. Contrast these with three clinically distinct abnormal end-range feels. Discuss capsular and noncapsular patterns.

Management of Orthopedic Conditions

Orthopedic Management of the Ankle, Foot, and Toes

Inversion ankle sprain
Deltoid ligament
Mechanical and functional instabilities
Subluxing peroneal tendons
Tendinitis
Plantar fasciitis
Lauge-Hansen
Distal tibia compression fractures (pilon fractures)
Calcaneal fractures
Talar fractures
Neuroma
Hallux valgus
Hammer toe
Mallet toe
Claw toe

MULTIPLE CHOICE

1. What percentage of all ankle sprains occurs to the lateral ligament complex?
   A. 50%
   B. 65%
   C. 95%
   D. 85%
2. What is the primary mechanism of injury to the lateral ligament complex of the ankle?
   A. Eversion, plantar flexion
   B. Plantar flexion, adduction, and eversion
   C. Inversion, plantar flexion, and adduction
   D. Dorsiflexion, abduction, and eversion
3. The anterior drawer test is used to clinically examine which ligaments of the ankle?
   A. Posterior talofibular ligament
   B. Anterior talofibular ligament

C. Fibulocalcaneal ligament
D. Deltoid ligament
E. All of the above

4. Which of the following represents potential pathologies that may be seen in conjunction with an inversion ankle sprain that is produced by inversion plantar flexion and adduction?
   A. Subluxing peroneal tendons
   B. Fracture of the base of the fifth metatarsal
   C. Malleolar fractures
   D. Sprains of the mid-foot
   E. All of the above
5. Using the injury classification model described by Leach, which of the following describes a second degree lateral ligament complex sprain of the ankle?
   A. The anterior talofibular ligament is completely torn
   B. The anterior talofibular ligament and fibulocalcaneal ligaments are completely torn
   C. All three ligaments are partially torn
   D. The anterior talofibular and fibulocalcaneal ligaments are partially torn
6. Which of the following best describes initial injury management of a grade II inversion ankle sprain?
   A. Short leg cast, crutches NWB
   B. RICE, crutches WBAT
   C. Ligament protection with semi-rigid external support, RICE, crutches, WBAT
   D. Cold whirlpool, crutches, NWB
7. Which of the following motions should be avoided during the acute and subacute phases of recovery from an inversion ankle sprain?
   A. Dorsiflexion
   B. Plantar flexion and inversion
   C. Eversion and dorsiflexion
   D. Plantar flexion and eversion
   E. All of the above

8. Deltoid ligament sprains of the ankle occur in what percentage of all ankle sprains?
   A. 10%
   B. 15%
   C. 7%
   D. 3% to 5%

9. Which of the following describe the mechanisms of injury for a deltoid ligament sprain of the ankle?
   A. Pronation and abduction
   B. Pronation and external rotation
   C. Supination and external rotation
   D. All of the above

10. What percentage of patients will suffer from chronic weakness, swelling, pain, and instability following either surgical repair or conservative treatment of inversion ankle sprains?
    A. 10% to 30%
    B. 15%
    C. 25%
    D. 3%

11. Mechanical instability is best defined as:
    A. Loss of joint proprioception
    B. Ligament laxity
    C. Subjective feeling of ankle giving way
    D. Mechanical block of normal joint motion

12. Functional instability is best described as:
    A. Ligament laxity
    B. Loss of muscular support
    C. Subjective sensation of joint instability
    D. Loss of gait proprioception

13. After surgery, if the peroneus brevis was used to stabilize the ankle, which of the following is(are) not allowed during the immediate postoperative period of recovery? (circle any that apply)
    A. Passive motions
    B. Active motions
    C. Manual resistance
    D. Eccentric contractions
    E. Plyometrics

14. Since functional ankle instabilities are classified as "giving way," a sense of instability without objective ligament laxity, the focus of rehabilitation is centered on:
    A. Pain relief
    B. Swelling reduction
    C. Proprioception drills and closed-chain resistance exercises
    D. Anaerobic power

15. In cases of acute subluxing peroneal tendons, the treatment of choice is:
    A. Surgery
    B. Immediate rehabilitation

C. Immobilization, NWB gait, and progressive rehabilitation
    D. Immobilization followed by full active ROM

16. Chronic subluxing peroneal tendons require:
    A. Immediate aggressive strengthening
    B. ROM exercises
    C. Casting followed by rehabilitation
    D. Surgery

17. In general, how many weeks of immobilization are required following surgery to correct chronic subluxing peroneal tendons?
    A. 2 weeks
    B. 6 weeks
    C. 16 weeks
    D. 9 weeks

18. Which of the following positions should be cautiously added following surgery to correct chronic subluxing peroneal tendons in order to allow for proper soft tissue and bone healing? (circle any that apply)
    A. Plantar flexion
    B. Inversion
    C. Dorsiflexion
    D. Eversion
    E. Terminal knee extension

19. Which of the following represents primary features of Achilles tendinitis?
    A. Muscular weakness
    B. Soft tissue swelling at the mid-portion of the calf
    C. Specific localized pain at the distal 1/3 of the tendon and the insertion on the calcaneus
    D. A palpable gap

20. The causes of Achilles tendinitis is (are): (circle any that apply)
    A. Sudden trauma (indirect)
    B. Direct trauma to the tendon
    C. Repetitive microtrauma
    D. Acute plantar flexion force
    E. Accumulative overload of the tendon

21. Which of the following represent(s) the most appropriate treatment for Achilles tendinitis? (circle any that apply)
    A. Surgery
    B. Cast immobilization
    C. NSAIDs, RICE
    D. Ultrasound, gentle ROM, progressive exercise
    E. NWB for 6 to 12 weeks

22. Which of the following describes the most common cause of a complete rupture of the Achilles tendon?
    A. Excessive, sudden plantar flexion
    B. Inversion

C. Eversion

D. Dorsiflexion

23. Where does the Achilles tendon rupture most commonly?

A. At the musculotendinous junction of the gastrocnemius

B. Mid-calf

C. 6 to 10 cm proximal to its insertion on the calcaneus

D. 3 to 4 cm proximal to its insertion on the calcaneus

24. Ruptures of the Achilles tendon occur most commonly to:

A. Women 20 to 50 years old

B. Men 15 to 20 years old

C. Women 40 to 60 years old

D. Men 20 to 50 years old

25. Clinically, to examine the affected leg for the presence of a ruptured Achilles tendon, the physical therapist will perform which test?

A. Anterior drawer test

B. Talar tilt test

C. Thompson test

D. Malleolar compression

26. Which of the following best describes how to perform the Thompson test?

A. Patient supine, knee flexed—squeeze the affected calf

B. Patient seated—knee flexed, squeeze the affected calf

C. Patient prone—knee extended, squeeze the affected calf

D. Patient prone—knee flexed, squeeze the affected calf

27. Which of the following generally describes the rate of re-rupture of the Achilles tendon if it is treated nonoperatively?

A. 10% to 20%

B. 8% to 39%

C. 50%

D. 5% to 20%

28. The duration of immobilization of a ruptured Achilles tendon treated nonoperatively is usually:

A. 4 to 6 weeks

B. 8 weeks

C. 16 weeks

D. 10 days

29. During the immobilization of a ruptured Achilles tendon, which of the following treatments are employed?

A. Quad and hamstring strengthening of the involved limb

B. Total body conditioning

C. UBE

D. Stationary cycle ergometer

E. All of the above

30. During nonoperative cast immobilization of a ruptured Achilles tendon, the affected ankle is placed in which position?

A. Dorsiflexion

B. Inversion

C. Eversion

D. Plantar flexion

31. When the cast is removed following nonoperative treatment of a ruptured Achilles tendon, the initial treatment will consist of: (circle any that apply)

A. Vigorous dorsiflexion exercise

B. Thermal agents, very gradual dorsiflexion range of motion

C. The use of a felt heel-lift to avoid excessive dorsiflexion

D. Gentle active plantar flexion range of motion

E. Ballistic stretching

32. The rehabilitation of postoperative repair of a ruptured Achilles tendon is:

A. Much faster than nonoperative treatment

B. Much slower than nonoperative treatment

C. Very similar to nonoperative rehabilitation

D. Much faster and does not follow the same criterion-based rehabilitation program as does operative rehabilitation

33. The organization and classification of ankle fractures described by Lauge-Hansen involve: (circle any that apply)

A. The direction of force

B. Specific patterns of injury

C. The age of the patient

D. The sex of the patient

E. All of the above

34. Ankle fractures include:

A. Lateral malleolar fractures

B. Medial malleolar fractures

C. Bi-malleolar fractures

D. Tri-malleolar fractures

E. All of the above

35. Generally, ankle fractures are treated with:

A. Crutch walking—WBAT

B. ORIF procedures

C. Compression wraps and NWB

D. Early active exercise

36. Throughout the duration of cast immobilization following surgery for an ankle fracture, which of the following can be prescribed?

A. Quad and hamstring strengthening for the involved limb

B. UBE

C. Total body conditioning

D. Single-leg stationary cycling

E. All of the above

37. Distal tibial compression fractures are also referred to as pilon fractures. These specific fractures occur from:

A. Rotational forces

B. Inversion forces

C. Axial or vertical loads

D. Eversion loads

E. All of the above

38. Because the mechanism of injury involves the articular surfaces of the distal tibia and the talus, weight-bearing activities following pilon fractures may be deferred for:

A. 8 weeks

B. 6 weeks

C. 10 weeks

D. 12 weeks

39. A common complication following a multi-fragmented compression fracture of the distal tibia is:

A. Severe vascular compromise

B. Neurological deficits

C. Secondary osteoarthritis

D. Rheumatoid arthritis

E. All of the above

40. The cornerstone in the recovery from a calcaneal fracture lies in regaining motion and strength of the:

A. Dorsiflexors

B. Inversion musculature

C. Eversion musculature

D. Plantar flexors

41. There are how many classifications of talar fractures?

A. 3

B. 4

C. 6

D. 5

42. A type II talar fracture with subtalar subluxation may result in? (circle any that apply)

A. Osteoarthritis

B. Neurovascular compromise

C. Avascular necrosis

D. Rheumatoid arthritis

E. Quad atrophy

43. Since talar fractures involve the articular surface, immobilization and NWB may last as long as:

A. 6 weeks

B. 3 months

C. 8 weeks

D. 4 weeks

44. Plantar fasciitis is caused by:

A. Acute plantar flexion

B. Acute dorsiflexion

C. Chronic traction on the plantar aponeurosis

D. Chronic inflammation of the flexor tendons

45. The treatment of plantar fasciitis can involve:

A. Surgery

B. Ice

C. NSAIDs

D. Stretching and strengthening exercises

E. All of the above

46. Which of the following are appropriate techniques to be used in the treatment of plantar fasciitis?

A. Nocturnal splints

B. Picking up marbles with the toes

C. Iontophoresis or phonophoresis

D. Toe extension stretches

E. All of the above

47. The most common location of Morton's neuroma is:

A. Medial and dorsal aspect of the foot

B. 3rd to 4th interspace

C. Plantar fascia

D. 2nd to 3rd interspace

48. Which of the following are various options for the treatment of Morton's neuroma? (circle any that apply)

A. Corticosteroid injections

B. Metatarsal pad

C. Cast immobilization

D. Change of footwear

E. Surgical excision

49. Following surgical correction of hallux valgus, the physical therapist will focus attention on: (circle any that apply)

A. Proper gait mechanics

B. Inversion strength of the ankle

C. Toe flexion and extension

D. Eversion strength of the ankle

E. Quad strength

50. Lesser toe deformities are generally made worse by:

A. Too much exercise

B. Kicking a ball

C. Improper shoe wear (narrow toe box)

D. High arch

SHORT ANSWER

51. Chronic instability may follow an inversion ankle sprain. Name the two types of instabilities associated with chronic ankle sprains.

52. Name the three major ligaments that represent the lateral ligament complex of the ankle.
53. Name the pathology shown in the figure.

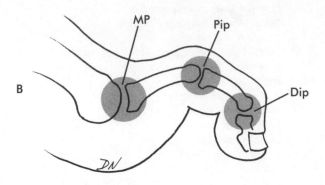

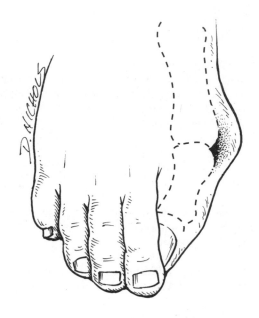

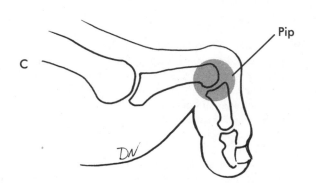

54. Match the following figures with the appropriate name of the deformity:

    Claw toe _____
    Hammer toe _____
    Mallet toe _____

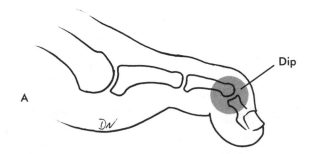

55. T or F   During the early recovery (acute phase) period of an inversion ankle sprain, it is imperative to instruct the patient to "write the alphabet" with the injured ankle.

56. T or F   Complete deltoid ligament sprains occur in combination with ankle fractures.

57. T or F   Mechanical instability may require surgery to stabilize the ankle.

58. T or F   Treatment for a ruptured Achilles tendon is always with surgery.

59. T or F   The loss of strength is less if the ruptured archilles tendon is treated nonsurgically.

60. T or F   The initial management of pilon fractures usually involves an ORIF procedure, external fixator, or skeletal traction.

61. T or F   In severe cases of plantar fasciitis, the physician may inject a local corticosteroid to reduce pain and swelling.

62. T or F   In cases of plantar fasciites where all conservative measures fail to bring significant results, the physician may elect to perform a fasciotomy or excision of a calcaneal exostosis.

63. T or F   Treatment of Morton's neuroma is always with surgical excision.

64. T or F   The removal of tight shoes may significantly reduce painful symptoms associated with hallux valgus.

65. T or F   Lesser toe deformities are characterized as either rigid or flexible.

66. T or F   Flexible toe deformities are most commonly corrected with surgery, whereas rigid toe deformities are corrected with conservative measures.

ESSAY QUESTIONS

Answer on a separate sheet of paper.
67. Identify common ligament injuries of the ankle.
68. Describe methods of management and rehabilitation of common ligament injuries to the ankle.
69. Identify and describe common tendon injuries to the ankle.
70. Outline and describe common methods of management and rehabilitation of tendon injuries to the ankle.

71. Identify common fractures of the foot and ankle.
72. Discuss common methods of management and rehabilitation of foot and ankle fractures.
73. Identify common toe deformities and describe methods of management and rehabilitation.
74. Describe common mobilization techniques for the ankle, foot, and toe.

CRITICAL THINKING APPLICATION

In small groups, develop two case studies: one related to a patient with a grade II anterior talofibular ligament sprain, the other, a patient with a displaced bimalleolar fracture.

In each case, develop a criterion-based rehabilitation program (critical pathway or critical mapping) that follows the maximum protection phase, moderate protection phase, and minimum protection phase concepts of progression. Be certain to apply your understanding of the mechanisms of soft tissue and bone healing and the three general phases of the inflammatory response, repair phase, and remodeling of tissues during each protective phase of recovery. Be specific in identifying the appropriate, safe, and effective use of agents to control pain and swelling. List exercises, activities, weight-bearing status, muscle contraction types, open- versus closed kinetic chain exercises, general physical conditioning, range of motion, cardiovascular fitness, balance-coordination-proprioception, and functional activities that are consistent with each phase of healing.

Orthopedic Management of the Knee

KEY TERMS

Anterior cruciate ligament (ACL)
Autograft
Allograft
Ligament-augmentation device (LAD)
Meniscus
Posterior cruciate ligament
Medial collateral ligament
Lateral collaterol ligament
Arthroscopy
Meniscal repair
Subtotal meniscectomy
Articular cartilage
Quadriceps angle (Q-angle)
Miserable malalignment syndrome
Supracondylar fractures
Tibial plateau fractures
Constrained
Nonconstrained
Osteotomy

MULTIPLE CHOICE

1. "A partial loss of ligament continuity, where a few ligament fibers may be completely torn and there is moderate pain, swelling, and some loss of joint function" is a description of what kind(s) of sprain? (circle any that apply)
   A. Grade I sprain
   B. Grade II sprain
   C. Grade III sprain
   D. Second degree sprain
2. External rotation, valgus stress, internal tibial rotation, and/or combined knee hyperextension defines mechanism of injury to which ligament?
   A. PCL
   B. MCL
   C. ACL
   D. LCL
3. Blood within the joint is referred to as:
   A. Swelling
   B. Effusion
   C. Hemarthrosis
   D. Blood clot
4. Arthrocentesis is:
   A. Joint arthrotomy
   B. A test for stability
   C. A test for vascular compromise
   D. Aspiration of fluid from a joint
5. Blood and fat seen on examination from arthrocentesis may represent:
   A. A meniscal tear and ligament tear
   B. An MCL sprain
   C. A ligament sprain and possible fracture
   D. Articular cartilage injury
6. It is important to recognize that the cruciate ligaments are:
   A. Extracapsular
   B. Rarely injured
   C. Always torn in isolation
   D. Intracapsular
7. If the MCL is sprained, there is usually:
   A. A great deal of swelling
   B. A tense hemarthrosis
   C. Minimal swelling
   D. Minimal pain and significant swelling
8. A clinically relevant ligament stability test used to examine the integrity of the ACL when the knee is flexed 25° to 30° is called:
   A. Anterior drawer test
   B. Valgus stress test

C. Pivot shift test

D. Lachman's test

9. An instrumented ligament stability testing device commonly used in the clinic to quantify anterior-posterior laxity is a:

A. PTS—Turbo 1000

B. KT 1000

C. Quantum 2000

D. A-P Tester

10. Tissue that is used from the body of the patient having surgery is called:

A. Allograft

B. Zenograft

C. Autograft

D. Gore-tex

11. The central one-third bone-patellar tendon-bone autograft surgical procedure describes a reconstruction of which ligament? (circle any that apply)

A. MCL

B. ACL

C. PCL

D. LCL

12. Which of the following tissues is(are) used for reconstruction of the ACL? (circle any that apply)

A. Gracilis tendon

B. Quadriceps tendon

C. Semitendinosus tendon

D. Fascia lata

E. Achilles tendon

13. An allograft refers to:

A. Synthetic tissue

B. Biologic tissue from another human body (cadaver)

C. Augmentation device

D. Prosthetic ligament

14. The major risks of surgery using an allograft are: (circle any that apply)

A. Disease transmission

B. Ineffective sterilization

C. Reduced vascular ingrowth

D. Rejection

E. Neurologic compromise

15. Which of the following tissues represents the strongest tissue available for autograft reconstruction of the ACL?

A. Gracilis tendon

B. Fascia lata

C. Bone-patellar tendon-bone

D. Quadriceps tendon

16. An extremely important point to remember is that the tissue used to surgically reconstruct the ACL goes through a process of:

A. Gradual vascular ingrowth during the first 6 to 8 weeks after surgery

B. Rapid collagen alignment, maturation, healing, and strength

C. Avascular necrosis in the first 6 to 8 weeks following surgery

D. Rapid strengthening then gradual loss of vascularity

17. While the newly placed graft is struggling to revascularize, it is essential to avoid: (circle any that apply)

A. Knee flexion

B. Terminal extension

C. Rotational forces

D. Anterior tibial translation forces

E. Ballistic closed kinetic chain exercises

18. Typically, scarring from the graft harvest site and suprapatellar pouch following an ACL reconstruction will inhibit: (circle any that apply)

A. Patellar mobility

B. Knee flexion

C. Weight bearing

D. Neurovascular status

E. Quad strength

19. During the maximum protection phase of recovery following ACL reconstruction, which of the following are allowed? (circle any that apply)

A. Passive terminal extension

B. Active short arc knee extensions

C. Isometric co-contraction of the quads and hams

D. Lightweight short arc knee extensions

E. Plyometrics

20. Which of the following exercises/exercise equipment would be appropriate for CKC exercises for a post-op ACL reconstruction patient 14 weeks after surgery? (circle any that apply)

A. Depth jumps

B. Stair steppers

C. Leg press

D. Treadmill

E. Horizontal bounding

21. Which of the following is a general criterion for the patient's readiness to progress from the moderate protection phase to the minimal protection phase after ACL reconstruction? (circle any that apply)

A. Full knee ROM

B. Squat with two times body weight

C. Perform single-leg plyometric hops

D. Be able to jog one-quarter mile

22. If the PCL is ruptured, the clinician performs an anterior and posterior drawer test, and the tibia is confirmed to translate or displace anteriorly, this exam should possibly be considered:

A. Positive for ACL tear
B. False negative
C. False positive for ACL tear
D. Negative PCL tear

23. A common denominator that exists between groups of patients treated surgically and those patients receiving conservative care for PCL tears is:
    A. Significant long-term dysfunction
    B. Vascular compromise
    C. Articular cartilage degeneration
    D. Meniscal tears

24. The most significant factor in rehabilitation of PCL injuries treated nonsurgically is:
    A. Gait dysfunction
    B. Quadriceps strengthening
    C. Hamstring strengthening
    D. Balance and coordination

25. Which of the following is not advocated during the maximum protection phase of recovery following an acute PCL tear treated surgically or non-operatively?
    A. Quadriceps strengthening
    B. Terminal passive extension
    C. Open kinetic chain resistance hamstring exercise
    D. Closed chain quadriceps exercise

26. A primary goal of recovery following PCL injuries is to strengthen:
    A. Hamstrings
    B. Quadriceps to exceed the strength of the non-injured limb
    C. Quadriceps equal to the non-injured limb
    D. Quadriceps and hamstrings equal to the non-injured limb

27. Common tissues used to reconstruct the PCL are: (circle any that apply)
    A. Achilles tendon
    B. Medial gastrocnemius tendon
    C. Semitendinosus tendon
    D. Patellar tendon
    E. Rotator cuff tendons

28. The most common ligament injury seen in the knee is:
    A. ACL
    B. MCL
    C. PCL
    D. LCL

29. What percentage of associated ligament injuries occurs in conjunction with a grade II MCL sprain?
    A. 20%
    B. 52%
    C. 75%
    D. 78%

30. The most common "unhappy triad" is:

A. PCL, ACL, LCL
B. ACL, MCL, lateral meniscus
C. ACL, MCL, medial meniscus
D. ACL, PCL, lateral meniscus

31. The MCL has direct anatomical attachment to the:
    A. Semitendinosus tendon
    B. Medial meniscus
    C. Medial gastrocnemius tendon
    D. Adductor magnus tendon

32. Which of the following is the most sensitive clinical exam to test the stability of the MCL?
    A. Lachman's test
    B. Anterior drawer
    C. Varus stress test
    D. Valgus stress test

33. The foundation of rehabilitation following MCL tears is to:
    A. Use NWB and cast immobilization
    B. Perform isometric exercises only during the maximum protection phase of recovery
    C. Use early protected motion
    D. Not use bracing and encourage early plyometric exercise

34. When prescribing hip adduction exercises following MCL injury, it is important to:
    A. Use 5 pounds or less of resistance
    B. Place the resistance distal to the joint line
    C. Place resistance proximal to the joint line
    D. Use 1 to 3 pounds of resistance

35. Which of the following highlight(s) the differences between rehabilitation and healing of the extracapsular MCL and intracapsular ACL and PCL? (circle any that apply)
    A. MCL has a high propensity to heal
    B. MCL has greater potential to heal because of its blood supply
    C. MCL is much stronger than the ACL
    D. Rehabilitation progresses much slower with MCL injuries
    E. Resistive knee flexion and extension exercises are prescribed earlier with MCL sprains as compared with ACL and PCL sprains

36. Which of the following may indicate a meniscal tear? (circle any that apply)
    A. History of twisting knee injury
    B. Hemarthrosis
    C. Valgus instability
    D. Swelling; locking of the knee
    E. Pain and "catching"

37. A test used to reproduce symptoms of torn meniscus is called:
    A. Smith test
    B. McMurray test

C. Pivot shift test

D. Lachman's test

38. A test used to determine if the meniscus is preventing knee extension is called:

A. Bounce home test

B. Tibial sag test

C. KT1000 test

D. Anterior drawer test

39. Which of the following surgical procedures will lead to limited early weight bearing, early limited full knee flexion, and generally slower advances with closed chain exercises in rehabilitation?

A. Total meniscectomy

B. Meniscal repair

C. Subtotal meniscectomy

D. Lateral release

40. Which of the following represent(s) long-term sequelae following total and subtotal meniscectomy? (circle any that apply)

A. Muscle atrophy

B. Joint space narrowing

C. Gait dysfunction

D. Degenerative arthritic changes

E. Neurological dysfunction

41. Following subtotal meniscectomy, weight-bearing status during the first week is usually:

A. NWB

B. 20% PWB

C. WBAT

D. 10% PWB

42. Which of the following describes the weight-bearing status following meniscal repair immediately post-op?

A. PWB

B. NWB progressing slowly to FWB at 4 to 6 week P-O

C. NWB progressing to FWB at 2 weeks P O

D. FWB

43. Closed kinetic chain resistance exercises, (such as leg press, squats, step-ups, and stair steppers, etc.) are generally not allowed for _____ following meniscal repair.

A. 3 to 4 weeks P-O

B. 4 to 6 weeks P-O

C. 8 weeks or longer P-O

D. 2 to 5 weeks P-O

44. Which of the following patellar positions is associated with a higher incidence of patellar instability?

A. Patella baja

B. Normal alignment

C. Patella alta

D. Patella infera

45. A line drawn from the anterior superior iliac spine (ASIS) through the center or axis of the patella and distally to the insertion of the patellar tendon on the tibial tubercle is called:

A. Varus deformity

B. Genu valgus

C. Q-angle

D. Genu recurvatum

46. Which of the following describe(s) the miserable malalignment syndrome? (circle any that apply)

A. External femoral rotation

B. Squinting patellae

C. External tibial torsion

D. Bayonet sign

E. Hypertrophy of the VMO

47. Which of the following are common recognizable signs and symptoms of anterior knee pain? (circle any that apply)

A. Crepitus

B. Laterally tracking patella

C. Pain

D. Vastus lateralis weakness

E. VMO weakness

48. The cornerstone in the rehabilitation of a painful laterally tracking patella is:

A. Hamstring stretching

B. Stretch lateral retinaculum

C. Strengthen quadriceps

D. Pain and swelling management

E. All of the above

49. In addition to strengthening the quadriceps (with anterior knee pain), which of the following muscle groups contribute to improving the appropriate line of pull on the patella?

A. Hip extensors

B. Hip adductors

C. Hip abductors

D. Hip flexors

E. All of the above

50. Which of the following is a proximal realignment surgical procedure for correction of anterior knee pain and a lateral tracking patella?

A. Elmslie-Trillat procedure

B. Howser procedure

C. Lateral retinacular release

D. Maquet procedure

51. Which of the following are surgical procedures used to reduce severe patellofemoral compression loads and significant lateral patellar subluxation by surgically realigning the distal extensor mechanism?

A. Distal-realignment procedures

B. Elmslie-Trillat procedure

C. "Radical" surgeries

D. Hauser procedure

E. All of the above

52. Which of the following is a procedure used to directly address retropatellar and femoral condyle articular cartilage degeneration? (circle any that apply)
    A. Perforation chondroplasty
    B. Abrasion arthroplasty
    C. Articular shaving
    D. Reefing
    E. Proximal realignment procedures

53. If a transverse fracture of the patella occurs, a complication of the proximal fracture segment may be:
    A. Malunion
    B. Nonunion
    C. Avascular necrosis
    D. Osteomalacia
    E. All of the above

54. Stabilization of displaced patellar fractures is best accomplished with:
    A. Rigid cast immobilization for 6 to 8 weeks
    B. Range limiting hinge-type knee brace for 6 to 8 weeks
    C. An ORIF procedure
    D. NWB for 4 to 6 weeks without immobilization

55. With tension-band wiring following a displaced patella fracture, the knee should be immobilized in which position?
    A. Terminal extension
    B. Knee flexion of 90°
    C. Range-limiting hinge brace set at 0° to 75°
    D. 20° of knee flexion

56. Distal femur fractures are classified as:
    A. Extraarticular
    B. Bicondylar
    C. Unicondylar
    D. Transverse supracondylar
    E. All of the above

57. Due to the proximity of the knee joint with a distal femur fracture, which of the following represents potential complications? (circle any that apply)
    A. Vascular injury
    B. Arthrofibrosis
    C. Adhesions
    D. Gait dysfunction
    E. Recurrent patellar subluxation

58. The purpose of a TKR (total knee replacement) is to: (circle any that apply)
    A. Correct deformity
    B. Improve function
    C. Eliminate or reduce pain
    D. Increase gait speed
    E. Reduce swelling

59. What is the most common age of persons with rheumatoid arthritis who undergo TKR?
    A. Less than 60 years old
    B. Less than 30 years old
    C. 75 years or older
    D. 60 to 75 years old

60. Which of the following is the goal of recovery following TKR?
    A. Relief of pain
    B. Restore mechanical axis of the knee
    C. Restore anatomical axis of the knee
    D. Provide adequate stability
    E. All of the above

61. A cruciate sparing implant is also referred to as: (circle any that apply)
    A. Conforming
    B. Constrained
    C. Nonconstrained
    D. Resurfacing implant
    E. Compression implant

62. Patellofemoral compression forces are estimated to be _____ times body weight while a person is walking on level surfaces.
    A. 1 to 1.5
    B. 2.5 to 3.0
    C. 5
    D. 4 to 5

63. What is the estimated patellofemoral compression forces while a person is ascending or descending stairs?
    A. 5 times body weight
    B. 3 to 4 times body weight
    C. 6 times body weight
    D. 2 to 3 times body weight

64. Which of the following describes the weight-bearing status of a patient following a TKR that is fixed with non-cemented prosthetic components?
    A. Limited weight bearing early with slow progression to full weight bearing by 12 weeks
    B. WBAT for 4 weeks, then full weight bearing
    C. NWB for 6 weeks, then progressing to full weight bearing by 8 weeks
    D. FWB by 6 weeks

65. What is the name of the surgical procedure performed for patients who have severe unicompartmental osteoarthritis of the knee?
    A. Howser procedure
    B. High tibial osteotomy
    C. Watson-Jones procedure
    D. Chondral shaving

66. A high tibial osteotomy attempts to:
    A. Lengthen the femur
    B. Lengthen the tibia
    C. Shorten the tibia
    D. Evenly distribute forces and compressive loads across the tibiofemoral joint

SHORT ANSWER

67. Which injury does this figure represent?

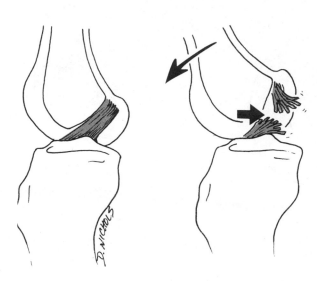

68. In the following figure, identify the ligament and name the exam being performed.

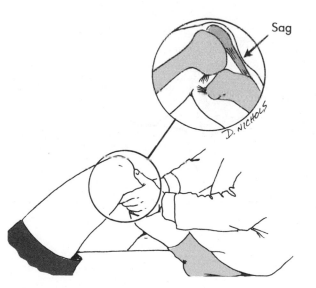

Sag

69. In the following figure, name the mechanism of injury and identify the torn structure:

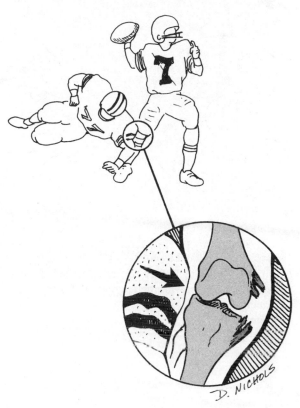

70. In the following figure, match the names of meniscal lesions with the appropriate diagrams. Select from these names: flap tear, longitudinal tear, parrot beak tear, bucket handle, radial tears.

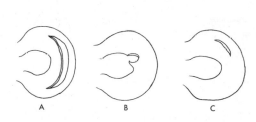

A   B   C

71. Match the following terms with the appropriate diagram: red-on-red zone, red-on-white zone, and white-on-white zone.

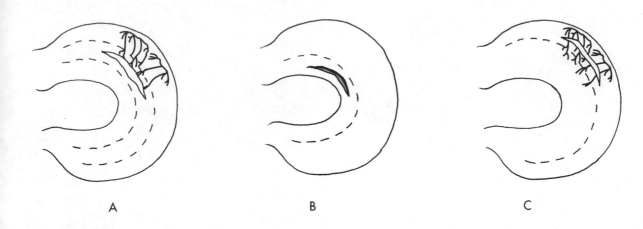

A   B   C

72. In the following figures, match the patellar reference description with the appropriate figure.
    Patella baja _____
    Patella alta _____
    Normal _____

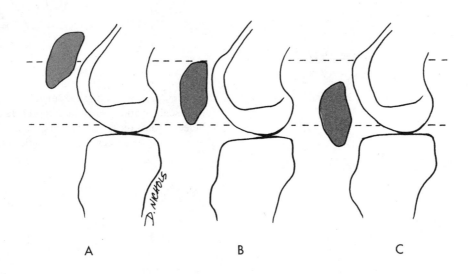

A   B   C

73. With supracondylar fractures there is the frequent occurrence of significant bleeding and tissue damage. List three early post-op management techniques to prevent or minimize knee flexion contractures.

74. In the following figure, name the general type of fracture and pattern of injury as well as identify the internal fixation devices used to secure the fracture fragments.

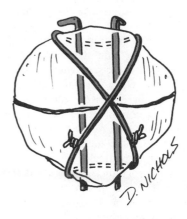

75. Name the two general types of implants used in a TKR.

TRUE/FALSE

76. T or F   The medial collateral ligament (MCL) is an extracapsular structure.
77. T or F   The concept of closed kinetic chain (CKC) exercise is not advocated during the moderate protection phase (from the seventh to the twelfth week after surgery) following ACL reconstruction.
78. T or F   When instructing a patient to perform a short arc leg press following a central one-third bone-patellar tendon-bone autograft, ACL reconstruction at 13 weeks post-op, it is not essential that the patient wear a brace.
79. T or F   Isolated posterior cruciate ligament (PCL) tears occur more frequently than ACL tears.
80. T or F   A grade I MCL sprain always occurs as an isolated injury.
81. T or F   Grade III MCL tears must always be treated surgically.
82. T or F   Apley's compression and distraction test is used to determine if the meniscus or ligament is injured.
83. T or F   Preservation of the load-bearing functions of the meniscus is the foundation for a subtotal meniscectomy.

84. T or F   Closed kinetic chain exercises are used during the fourth to the eighth post-operative week following sub-total meniscectomy.
85. T or F   Full knee range of motion is allowed following meniscal repairs as soon as the patient can tolerate.
86. T or F   Excessive hamstring tightness may contribute to increased patellofemoral compression.
87. T or F   In the case of a lateral retinacular release without VMO advancement, it is generally appropriate to encourage early post-operative knee flexion range of motion in order to keep the deep surgically cut tissues "open."
88. T or F   In cases where a lateral retinacular release was performed in addition to a VMO advancement, early quadriceps strengthening and knee flexion must be encouraged.
89. T or F   The treatment of nondisplaced patellar fractures is with rigid immobilization in terminal extension.
90. T or F   Following immobilization of a nondisplaced patellar fracture, early quadriceps strengthening and full knee flexion range of motion is encouraged.
91. T or F   Nondisplaced tibial plateau fractures are always treated with an ORIF procedure.
92. T or F   The method of implant fixation of patellar, femoral, or tibial components of a TKR has no direct impact on immediate postoperative rehabilitation.
93. T or F   Prosthetic implant fixation of the components of a TKR can be achieved in two ways: bone cement (PMMA), or a porous-coated, cementless prosthesis.
94. T or F   With severe osteoarthritis of the knee, the most common compartment affected is the lateral knee joint compartment, which results in a valgus deformity.

ESSAY QUESTIONS

Answer on a separate sheet of paper.
95. Identify common ligament injuries of the knee.
96. Discuss common methods of management and rehabilitation of common ligament injuries of the knee.
97. Identify and describe common meniscal injuries of the knee.
98. Discuss common methods of management and rehabilitation of meniscal injuries of the knee.

99. Identify and describe common patellofemoral pathologies of the knee.
100. Describe common methods of management and rehabilitation of patellofemoral disease pathologies of the knee.
101. Identify and describe common fractures of the patella, supracondylar femur fractures, and proximal tibia fractures.
102. Describe common methods of management and rehabilitation of fractures about the knee.
103. Identify and describe methods of management and rehabilitation following knee arthroplasty and high tibial osteotomy.
104. Describe common mobilization techniques for the knee.

CRITICAL THINKING APPLICATION

You are treating a patient with a diagnosis of postoperative ACL reconstruction using the central one-third bone-patellar tendon-bone autograft. In addition, the patient also had a repair of the medical meniscus. It is 1 week after surgery. Develop a continuum of progressive rehabilitation (critical-pathway, -criterion-based rehab program) that follows the maximum protection phase, moderate protection phase, and minimum protection phase concept of recovery. Based on your knowledge of soft tissue injury and repair, be certain your program of rehabilitation is consistent with the overlapping phases of injury repair.

For each phase of healing, identify and recommend appropriate agents for pain and swelling management. For each phase, list exercises, range of motion, muscle contraction types, weight-bearing status, open- and closed-kinetic chain exercises, cardiovascular fitness, general physical conditioning, balance-coordination-proprioception drills, and return to functional activities.

What effect does the meniscal repair have on the development of this particular rehabilitation program? How would this program be different if the meniscus were not injured? What modifications in this program would be necessary if the ACL were not injured and just the meniscus was repaired?

Orthopedic Management of the Hip and Pelvis

KEY TERMS

Avascular necrosis (AVN)
Open reduction and internal fixation (ORIF)
Degenerative joint disease (DJD)
Proximal femoral intertrochanteric osteotomy
Hemi-arthroplasty
Total hip replacement (THR)
Total hip precautions
Legg-Calvé-Perthes (LCP) disease
Trochanteric Bursitis
Strains
Contusions

MULTIPLE CHOICE

1. Which of the following represent(s) the most significant complication following hip fracture? (circle any that apply)
   A. Avascular necrosis
   B. Muscular atrophy
   C. Venous thrombosis
   D. Endurance
   E. Gait dysfunction
2. Avascular necrosis may occur following hip fracture in approximately what percentage of patients?
   A. 10% to 20%
   B. 50% to 60%
   C. 65% to 85%
   D. 5% to 15%
3. Which of the following describe(s) clinical complications noted with subtrochanteric fractures of the hip? (circle any that apply)
   A. Muscular atrophy
   B. Malunion
   C. Delayed union

   D. Nonunion
   E. Decreased hip abduction
4. Without prophylactic medications, what percentage of patients may develop thrombosis following hip surgery?
   A. 20%
   B. 10% to 15%
   C. 40% to 90%
   D. 5% to 10%
5. During the first 6 to 8 weeks following a hip fracture secured with an ORIF procedure, which of the following exercises must be avoided?
   A. Quad sets
   B. Heel slides
   C. Supine straight-leg raises
   D. Gluteal sets
6. During the early recovery phase of healing following a hip fracture (6 to 8 weeks), which of the following exercises must be avoided?
   A. Knee flexion with hip flexion
   B. Rotary or diagonal hip patterns of movement
   C. Knee flexion
   D. Hip extension
   E. All of the above
7. Which of the following procedures is used in cases of femoral head osteonecrosis or severe femoral head fractures?
   A. Femoral osteotomy
   B. Hemiarthroplasty
   C. Tibial osteotomy
   D. Plate and screw fixation
8. Which of the following is(are) generally the goal(s) following hemiarthroplasty of the hip?
   A. Increase muscle size
   B. Improve neuromuscular endurance
   C. Reduce pain and improve function
   D. Increase hip range of motion

9. Which of the following are indications for total hip replacement (THR)?
   A. Rheumatoid arthritis
   B. Osteoarthritis
   C. Severe fractures
   D. Osteonecrosis
   E. All of the above

10. Which of the following represents one of the more common complications of total hip arthroplasty using a noncemented femoral stem component?
    A. Quadriceps weakness
    B. Quadriceps atrophy
    C. Persistent thigh pain and related antalgic gait
    D. Reduced hip range of motion

11. Following THR, which of the following is the most significant complication with the highest mortality rate?
    A. Malunion
    B. Thromboembolic disease
    C. Avascular necrosis
    D. Nonunion

12. Postoperative dislocation of the hip following THR, according to Miller, is a clinically significant complication that occurs in approximately:
    A. 10% of patients
    B. 50% of patients
    C. 15% of patients
    D. 1% to 4% of patients

13. Which of the following generally describe(s) universal hip precautions after THR? (circle any that apply)
    A. Avoid hip adduction
    B. Avoid external rotation
    C. Avoid hip flexion greater than 90°
    D. Avoid hip internal rotation
    E. Avoid knee flexion greater than 80°

14. Which of the following are appropriate exercises during the immediate postoperative recovery following a THR? (circle any that apply)
    A. Partial squats
    B. Short arc step-ups
    C. Quad sets
    D. Gluteal isometrics
    E. Hamstring sets

15. With a cemented hip prosthesis, how soon can closed kinetic chain functional activities be initiated?
    A. As soon as pain allows
    B. When hip range of motion improves
    C. Between 3 and 8 weeks post-op and with increased weight-bearing orders by the physician
    D. Between 8 and 10 weeks post-op

16. A noninflammatory, self-limiting syndrome in which the femoral head becomes flattened at the weight-bearing surface as a result of disruption of the blood supply to the femoral head in the growing child is called: (circle any that apply)
    A. Coxa plana
    B. Avascular necrosis
    C. Legg-Calvé-Perthes disease
    D. Osteoporosis
    E. Capsulitis

17. In cases of acute hamstring strain, which position would provide the greatest support at night?
    A. Supine knee extended
    B. Prone knee extended
    C. Supine knee flexed with pillow for support
    D. Sidelying
    E. All of the above

18. What is a "hip pointer"?
    A. A contusion to the ischial tuberosity
    B. A contusion of the rectus femoris
    C. A contusion of the iliac crest
    D. An indirect strain of the rectus femoris

19. In general, stable pelvic fractures are treated with: (circle any that apply)
    A. With an ORIF procedure
    B. Protected weight bearing
    C. Bed rest
    D. Progressive motion
    E. Closed chain eccentric exercise

20. Unstable pelvic fractures are considered: (circle any that apply)
    A. Easily treated
    B. Not complicated
    C. Severe and potentially life-threatening
    D. Not medically challenging
    E. Common pediatric fractures

21. Due to the fragile vascular and potentially unstable hemodynamic nature of significant pelvic fractures, weight bearing of any kind is deferred for:
    A. 2 to 4 weeks
    B. 3 to 5 weeks
    C. 8 weeks or longer
    D. 4 to 6 weeks

22. Fractures of the acetabulum are significant because: (circle any that apply)
    A. They are always unstable
    B. The acetabulum is an articular weight-bearing surface
    C. Acetabular fractures can result in osteoarthritis of the hip
    D. These injuries always lead to a THR
    E. They are usually treated with an ORIF procedure

SHORT ANSWER

23. In the following figure, name the type of injury.

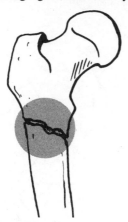

24. In the following figure, name the type of injury.

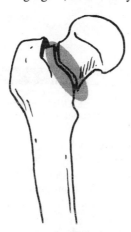

25. In the following figure, name the type of injury.

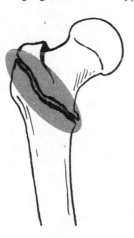

26. In the following figure, name the soft tissue injury.

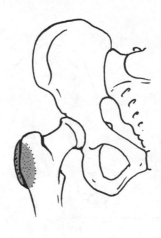

27. In the following figure, name the soft tissue injury.

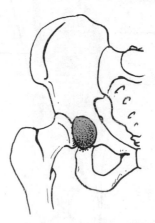

28. In the following figure, name the soft tissue injury.

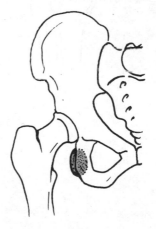

29. In the following figure, label each muscle.

30. In the following figure, identify the fracture type and location of injury.

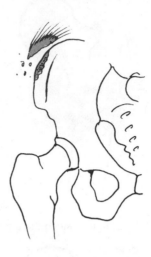

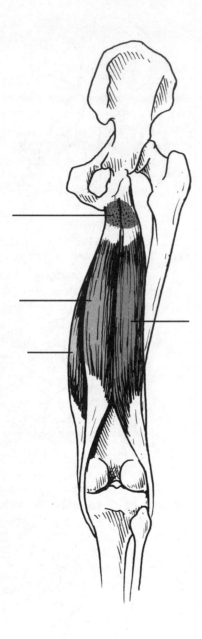

31. T or F   Hip fractures represent the most common acute orthopedic injury in the geriatric population.

32. T or F   The subtrochanteric area of the hip is prone to large biomechanical stresses, which can lead to loosening of various internal fixation devices.

33. T or F   The treatment of a fractured greater trochanter of the hip will always be with an ORIF procedure.

34. T or F   The general progression of weight-bearing status following hip fractures will usually parallel the rate of bone healing.

35. T or F   The method of fixation of various prosthetic hip components will have a direct impact on the short-term and long-term course of rehabilitation following hip arthroplasty.

36. T or F   Noncemented biologic tissue ingrowth prostheses will require longer periods of limited weight bearing than cemented prosthetic hip components.

37. T or F   It is clinically significant that the simultaneous performance of hip flexion, internal rotation, and adduction be avoided for up to 4 months after THR surgery.

38. T or F   It is appropriate to actively encourage full knee extension following a hamstring strain during the first 3 weeks following injury.

39. T or F   Unstable pelvic fractures are generally defined as either rotationally unstable but vertically stable, or rotationally and vertically unstable.

40. T or F   Closed kinetic chain exercises are advocated during the early healing phases of recovery following acetabular fractures.

ESSAY QUESTIONS

Answer on a separate sheet of paper.
41. Identify common hip fractures.
42. Outline and discuss common methods of management and rehabilitation of common hip fractures.
43. Identify and describe common methods of management and rehabilitation following hip arthroplasty.
44. Identify and describe common soft tissue injuries of the hip.
45. Outline and describe common methods of management and rehabilitation of soft tissue injuries of the hip.
46. Identify common fractures of the pelvis and the hip.
47. Discuss methods of management and rehabilitation for fractures of the pelvis and acetabulum.

48. Describe common mobilization techniques for the hip.

CRITICAL THINKING APPLICATION

You are treating two patients; one patient has a subtrochanteric hip fracture with an ORIF, the other patient has a total hip arthroplasty in which the prosthetic components are secured (fixed) with cement.

In small groups, contrast the differences in rehabilitation progression, weight-bearing status, complications, and precautions related to these two cases. Specifically, define and contrast hip precautions related to hip fractures and hip arthroplasty. Identify and list appropriate range-of-motion exercises, muscle contraction types, weight-bearing status, general physical conditioning, cardiovascular fitness, open and closed kinetic chain activities, balance-coordination-proprioception drills and a progressive return to function consistent with your understanding of soft tissue and bone healing. Does the method of prosthetic hip component fixation affect your recommendations related to motion, strength, and weight-bearing status? Clearly identify all complications related to fractures and surgery of the hip.

Orthopedic Management of the Lumbar, Thoracic, and Cervical Spine

MULTIPLE CHOICE

1. The second leading cause of all physician visits in the United States is:
   A. The common cold
   B. Knee sprains
   C. Ankle sprains
   D. Lumbar spine injuries

2. When the lumbar spine moves from a position of flexion into extension, the nucleus tends to displace in which direction?
   A. Anteriorly
   B. Posteriorly
   C. Laterally
   D. Diagonally

3. When the lumbar spine moves from a position of extension into flexion, the nucleus tends to displace in which direction?
   A. Laterally
   B. Diagonally
   C. Posteriorly
   D. Arteriorly

4. Which of the following accurately describe(s) key features of basic lifting mechanics? (circle any that apply)
   A. Keep a wide base of support
   B. Keep the object lifted away from the body
   C. Maintain a lordotic posture
   D. Use the legs to lift
   E. Exhale on the lift phase

5. Muscular strains of the lumbar spine are common and occur from:
   A. Sudden muscular contractions
   B. Rapid stretching
   C. Torque
   D. Eccentric loading
   E. All of the above

6. Walking has been shown to be an effective exercise for the treatment of lumbar muscle strain because walking:
   A. Stimulates circulation
   B. Enhances cardiovascular and cardiorespiratory fitness

C. Stimulates the mechanoreceptor system

D. Improves coordination and strength

E. All of the above

7. A generalized phase I or acute management of lumbar sprains or strains will focus on: (circle any that apply)

A. Immediate functional activities

B. Pain control

C. Swelling management

D. Restricted motions

E. Combined flexion and rotation motions

8. If the posterior longitudinal ligament of the lumbar spine is sprained, which position(s) should be avoided during the maximum protection phase?

A. Lateral flexion

B. Extension

C. Flexion

D. Rotation

E. All of the above

9. Which of the following describes an extruded disc?

A. Nucleus is free in the canal

B. Nucleus bulges against annulus

C. Nucleus extends through the annulus, but the nuclear material is contained by the posterior longitudinal ligament

D. Nucleus is intact, but the annulus is ruptured

10. Herniated nucleus pulposus (HNP) is a disease that primarily affects which age group?

A. Young adults only

B. Adults more than 50 years old only

C. Elderly, more than 70 years old

D. Young to middle-age adults

11. Which of the following describes back pain that is aggravated by activity and relieved by rest?

A. Neurogenic pain

B. Vascular pain

C. Spondylogenic pain

D. Viscerogenic pain

12. Which of the following describes radicular signs related to HNP?

A. Numbness

B. Radiating pain

C. Posterior thigh pain

D. Paresthesias radiating distally below the knee

E. All of the above

13. Which of the following is(are) the objective(s) for management of HNP?

A. Protection from unwanted forces

B. Increased muscular strength, flexibility, endurance

C. Enhanced awareness and performance of proper body mechanics

D. Pain and swelling relief

E. All of the above

14. Which of the following describes the most common surgical procedure used to treat HNP?

A. Laminotomy with decompression discectomy

B. Microsurgical discectomy

C. Percutaneous discectomy

D. Multisegment fusion

15. Which of the following describe(s) Williams exercises? (circle any that apply)

A. Pelvic tilt

B. Single knee to chest

C. Prone extension

D. Partial direct sit-ups

E. Lateral trunk flexion

16. Studies have shown that isometric lumbar training and testing can produce increases of up to _____ in strength. (circle any that apply)

A. 50%

B. 80%

C. 100%

D. Several thousand percent

E. 20% to 30%

17. Which of the following describes potential uses for lumbar spine testing procedures?

A. Measure progress objectively

B. Medicolegal use

C. Research

D. Job screening and worksite evaluations

E. All of the above

18. Which of the following describe(s) contraindications for static or dynamic lumbar strength testing? (circle any that apply)

A. Chronic pain

B. Unstable fractures

C. Acute injury

D. Sequestrated disc

E. Fatigue

19. Which of the following is an ergonomic risk factor identified in the administration of a functional capacity evaluation (FCE)?

A. Height

B. Amount of weight that can be lifted

C. How often load is lifted

D. How high load is lifted

E. All of the above

20. A narrowing of the spinal canal constricting and compressing nerve roots that produces symptoms of neurogenic or spinal claudication is called:

A. HNP

B. Sequestrated disc

C. Spondylolysis
D. Spinal stenosis
21. Spinal stenosis occurs:
    A. In males twice as often as females
    B. In females more often than males
    C. In young males
    D. In older females more often than older males
22. Spinal stenosis is most commonly acquired:
    A. By overt trauma
    B. By repetitive motion
    C. By degenerative arthritic changes
    D. Due to weakness of the paraspinal musculature
23. The patient with spinal stenosis will frequently complain of increased symptoms with:
    A. Lumbar extension
    B. Lumbar flexion
    C. Ambulating in flexed lumbar posture
    D. Pelvic tilts
    E. All of the above
24. A forward slippage of one superior vertebra over an inferior vertebra (usually L_4-L_5 or L_5-S_1) is called:
    A. Spondylolysis
    B. Stenosis
    C. Spinal claudication
    D. Spondylolisthesis
25. The most common type or classification of spondylolisthesis is:
    A. Congenital
    B. Isthmic
    C. Degenerative
    D. Traumatic
26. A grade III spondylolisthesis is defined as forward slippage of:
    A. 25% to 50%
    B. 0% to 25%
    C. 50% to 75%
    D. 75% to 100%
27. Compression fractures of the spine can commonly occur in the elderly with osteoporosis from:
    A. High force flexion
    B. Ballistic extension
    C. Benign daily activities
    D. High force rotation
    E. All of the above
28. Which of the following motions should be avoided during the acute and subacute phases following compression fractures?
    A. Flexion
    B. Extension
    C. Rotation
    D. Lateral flexion
    E. All of the above

29. What is the incidence (percentage of the population) of thoracic disc herniations?
    A. 7%
    B. 10%
    C. 0.3%
    D. 2%
30. The segments most commonly involved with thoracic disc herniations are:
    A. Between the first and fifth vertebrae
    B. Between the ninth and twelfth vertebrae
    C. Between the second and fourth vertebrae
    D. All segments equally
31. An increase in the thoracic posterior convexity is defined as:
    A. Lordosis
    B. Kyphosis
    C. Scoliosis
    D. Osteoporosis
32. In general, the treatment of kyphosis will focus on:
    A. Postural awareness
    B. Stretching the pectorals
    C. Thoracic extension strengthening
    D. Strengthening the scapular retractors
    E. All of the above
33. With structural scoliosis the physical therapist assistant will note that:
    A. With extension, the identified curve does not decrease
    B. With lateral flexion, the curve dissipates
    C. With trunk flexion, the curve does not decrease
    D. With trunk flexion, the curve dissipates
34. Which of the following represents significant clinical features of scoliosis with thoracic curves greater than 65°?
    A. Pain
    B. Neurologic symptoms
    C. Decreased cardiopulmonary function
    D. Cosmetic
    E. All of the above
35. The effective use of therapeutic exercise for the treatment of scoliosis is designed to:
    A. Reduce pain
    B. Increase motion
    C. Enhance strength
    D. Promote function
    E. All of the above
36. Which of the following is a fundamental principle in the care of idiopathic scoliosis?
    A. Develop anaerobic power
    B. Develop thoracic and lumbar extension strength

C. Stretch the concave side of the curve, while simultaneously strengthening the convex side of the curve

D. Develop trunk flexion strength

37. In experimental studies, which of the following structures have been identified as being involved with cervical hyperextension-type automobile accidents?
A. Sternocleidomastoid
B. Anterior longitudinal ligament
C. Longissimus coli muscle
D. Separation of cartilaginous end-plate of the intervertebral disc
E. All of the above

38. Similarly, hyperflexion injuries of the cervical spine can result in: (circle any that apply)
A. Tears of the anterior longitudinal ligaments
B. Tears of the ligamentum nuchae
C. Intervertebral disc injury
D. Tears of the posterior longitudinal ligament
E. Tears of the anterior deltoid

39. Initial strengthening of the cervical spine following a strain and/or sprain is usually accomplished by introducing:
A. Manually applied eccentric contractions
B. Submaximal concentric muscle contractions
C. Submaximal isometric contractions
D. Maximal, multiangle isometrics

40. Which of the following represents one of the more commonly recognized malalignment syndromes of the cervical spine?
A. Lateral flexion malalignment
B. Cervical extension malalignment
C. Forward head posture
D. Cervical rotation malalignment

41. To correct for a forward head posture, a commonly applied series of exercises is: (circle any that apply)
A. Cervical flexion isometrics
B. Axial extension exercises
C. Head extension isometrics
D. Cervical retraction exercises
E. All of the above

42. Proximal compression of the subclavian artery and vein as well as the brachial plexus are probable neurovascular structures involved with:
A. Volkmann's ischemic contracture
B. Carpal tunnel syndrome
C. Thoracic outlet syndrome
D. De Quervain's tenosynovitis

43. Which of the following is a symptom of neurovascular tissue compression?
A. Radicular pain
B. Weakness

C. Numbness
D. Tingling
E. All of the above

44. Which of the following exercises are most appropriate for the care of thoracic outlet syndrome?
A. Thoracic flexion exercises
B. Lateral cervical flexion exercises
C. Thoracic extension, scapular retraction, and pectoral stretching
D. Cervical flexion exercises

SHORT ANSWER

45. Match the following list of percentages relating to intradiscal pressure with the appropriate and corresponding body position.
100%   supine (knees flexed)
75%   standing
35%   bending forward
25%   sidelying
275%   supine

46. List the five *Ls* of lifting, as described by O'Sullivan, Ellis, and Makofsky.

47. In the following figure, identify the category of lumbar disc injury.

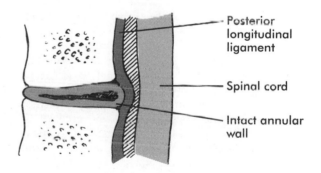

Posterior longitudinal ligament

Spinal cord

Intact annular wall

48. In the following figure, identify the category of lumbar disc injury.

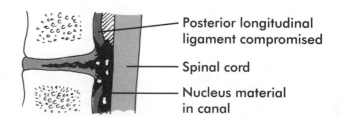

Posterior longitudinal ligament compromised

Spinal cord

Nucleus material in canal

TRUE/FALSE

49. T or F   The intervertebral lumbar disc is essentially avascular and aneural except for the periphery of the annulus, which is innervated.

50. T or F   Ligamentous sprains of the lumbar spine can occur from either sudden violent force or repeated stress.

51. T or F   It is essential that all cases of HNP be treated with lumbar extension postures.

52. T or F   Manual muscle testing is the most effective way to quantify lumbar muscle strength and performance.

53. T or F   Lumbar extension exercises are advocated for spondylolisthesis.

54. T or F   Osteoporosis, which can lead to multilevel thoracic compression fractures, can cause anterior wedging of the segments, which in turn creates the kyphotic curve.

55. T or F   Scoliosis refers to a lateral curvature of the lumbar vertebrae.

56. T or F   Generally, scoliosis can be categorized as either structural or nonstructural.

57. T or F   With nonstructural scoliosis, positional changes result in a decrease in the curvature.

58. T or F   Therapeutic exercise (by itself) is intended to halt the progression of scoliosis as well as correct resultant deformity.

59. T or F   The use of bracing in the treatment of scoliosis is intended to halt the progression of the curve and is not identified as effective in correcting cosmetic deformity.

60. T or F   Axial stretching (trunk elongation) is not advocated for the treatment of scoliosis.

61. T or F   Cervical spondylosis is an acute cervical disc disorder.

ESSAY QUESTIONS

Answer on a separate sheet of paper.

62. Outline and describe the basic mechanics of the lumbar spine.

63. Discuss and apply the principles of the fundamental mechanics of lifting.

64. Identify common sprains and strains of the lumbar spine.

65. Discuss common methods of management and rehabilitation of lumbar spine sprains and strains.

66. Identify and describe injuries to the lumbar intervertebral disc.

67. Discuss methods of management and rehabilitation for injuries to the lumbar intervertebral disc.

68. Define and describe methods of quantifying back strength.

69. Define and describe components of the back school model.

70. Define ergonomic and functional capacity evaluations.

71. Define spinal stenosis and describe methods of management and rehabilitation.

72. Define and contrast the terms *spondylosis* and *spondylolisthesis*.

73. Describe methods of management and rehabilitation for spondylolysis and spondylolisthesis.

74. Identify common lumbar and thoracic spine fractures.

75. Define kyphosis, lordosis, and scoliosis.

76. Identify and describe methods of management and rehabilitation for kyphosis and scoliosis.

77. Identify and describe common cervical spine injuries and discuss methods of management and rehabilitation.

CRITICAL THINKING APPLICATION

Based on your knowledge and understanding of the mechanisms of the lumbar spine and the healing mechanisms of soft tissue and bone, develop a comprehensive rehabilitation program (critical pathway, criterion-based rehab program) for a patient with an extruded disc at L_4-L_5. Which activities would you recommend during the acute phase of recovery? Which positions would you encourage and which would you discourage? Identify and list four general objectives for the care of an HNP. During each phase of recovery, recommend specific restrictions, agents to aid in pain and swelling management, alterations in body mechanics, flexibility exercises, aerobic fitness, strength training, and balance and proprioception drills. Assuming this patient is a manual laborer who is required to lift boxes from the floor and place them on a truck, what specific ergonomic modifications would you recommend? Is back school an option? If so, list the components of a comprehensive back school program. If this patient sits at a desk all day, what ergonomic design modifications would you recommend?

Orthopedic Management of the Shoulder

KEY TERMS

Subacromial rotator cuff impingement
Scapular stabilization exercises
Codman's pendulum exercises
Dislocation
Subluxation
Bankart lesion
Hill-Sachs lesion
TUBS
AMBRI
Capsulitis
Acromioclavicular (A-C) joint
Open reduction and internal fixation (ORIF)

MULTIPLE CHOICE

1. Mechanical compression of the rotator cuff tendons, primarily the supraspinatus tendon, as they pass under the coracoacromial ligament between the coracoid and the acromion process is termed:
   A. Secondary impingement
   B. Thoracic outlet syndrome
   C. Primary impingement
   D. Bicipital tendinitis
2. Which of the following is the most common structure involved with impingement of the shoulder?
   A. Subscapularis tendon
   B. Infraspinatus tendon
   C. Supraspinatus tendon
   D. Biceps tendon
3. An area just proximal to the insertion of the supraspinatus on the greater tuberosity is (are): (circle any that apply)

A. Hypervascular
B. The watershed zone
C. Hypovascular
D. The critical zone
E. Neer's zone

4. Which of the following describe(s) Neer's stage II impingement? (circle any that apply)
   A. Is a reversible lesion
   B. Occurs to persons 25 to 40 years of age
   C. Is characterized by tendon degeneration
   D. Is fibrosis of the subacromial tissues
   E. Is an irreversible lesion
5. Which of the following describe(s) rotator cuff impingement signs? (circle any that apply)
   A. Pain with shoulder abduction between 60° and 120°
   B. Pain with forward flexion
   C. Pain with shoulder extension
   D. Pain with forced internal rotation with the affected arm abducted to 90°
   E. Pain with elbow flexion
6. Which of the following muscles must be strengthened prior to addressing specific rotator cuff weakness in the presence of secondary rotator cuff impingement? (circle any that apply)
   A. Pectorals
   B. Serratus anterior
   C. Latissimus dorsi
   D. Rhomboids
   E. Middle deltoid
7. A general, comprehensive rehabilitation plan for treatment of rotator cuff impingement during early recovery stage includes:
   A. Scapular stabilization exercises
   B. Repetitive overhead lifting
   C. Specific rotator cuff strengthening

D. Pectoral strengthening

E. None of the above

8. ADL modifications and exercise modifications in the presence of subacromial rotator cuff impingement include:

A. Avoid forward flexion above 30°

B. Limit abduction below 80° or 90°

C. Avoid abduction entirely

D. Avoid internal rotation

E. All of the above

9. Studies demonstrate the highest electromyographic activity for strengthening the supraspinatus, infraspinatus, subscapularis, deltoid, latissimus dorsi, and pectorals involves: (circle any that apply)

A. Scaption

B. Prone horizontal abduction with external rotation

C. Elbow extension

D. Arm elevation in sagittal plane

E. Scapular elevation

10. Rowing exercises, scapular plane elevation (scaption), press-ups, and push-ups with a plus define:

A. Specific rotator cuff exercise

B. Specific throwing exercises

C. Scapular stabilization exercises

D. Specific exercises for scoliosis

11. Which of the following describe(s) the most common positions that may induce anterior glenohumeral subluxation or dislocation? (circle any that apply)

A. Arm abducted

B. Internal rotation

C. Shoulder extension

D. External rotation

E. Shoulder adduction

12. Which is the most commonly dislocated joint in the body?

A. Knee

B. Elbow

C. Shoulder

D. Hip

13. This injury occurs as a result of glenohumeral dislocation and is defined as an avulsion of the capsule and glenoid labrum off of the anterior rim of the glenoid.

A. Rotator cuff tear

B. Bankart lesion

C. Hill-Sachs lesion

D. Subacromial impingement

14. The initial nonoperative management of glenohumeral instability calls for a period of immobilization lasting:

A. 2 weeks

B. More than 8 weeks

C. Up to 6 weeks

D. 3 weeks

15. Which of the following exercises are prescribed for the affected immobilized shoulder with acute anterior glenohumeral dislocation?

A. Full range-of-motion concentric exercise

B. Limited range of motion eccentric exercises

C. Submaximal isometrics

D. Isokinetic exercise

E. All of the above

16. For up to 3 months or longer after removal of the sling, which motions need to be limited following anterior glenohumeral dislocation?

A. Flexion and extension

B. Internal and external rotation

C. Abduction and external rotation

D. Extension and internal rotation

17. Which of the following is the appropriate ratio of motion between the scapula and glenohumeral joint after the first 30° of glenohumeral flexion or abduction?

A. 3:1

B. 2:2

C. 2:1

D. 1:1

18. Which of the following represent(s) general categories of surgical stabilization procedures used for glenohumeral instability? (circle any that apply)

A. Surgical repairs of Bankart lesions

B. Surgical repairs of Hill-Sachs lesions

C. Bone block and coracoid process transfers

D. Procedures to limit external rotation

E. Surgical procedures to limit internal rotation

19. Which of the following describes adhesive capsulitis, or "frozen shoulder"?

A. Pain

B. Reduced range of motion

C. Inflamed capsule

D. Fibrous synovial adhesions

E. All of the above

20. Adhesive capsulitis commonly affects:

A. Men 40 to 60 years old

B. Women 20 to 30 years old

C. Women 40 to 60 years old

D. Men 60 years and older

21. Which of the following is(are) the classifications of adhesive capsulitis? (circle any that apply)

A. Tertiary

B. Resistant

C. Secondary

D. Primary

E. Profound

22. Adhesive capsulitis, which occurs spontaneously from unknown causes, is referred to as:
    A. Tertiary
    B. Primary adhesive capsulitis
    C. Secondary adhesive capsulitis
    D. Resistant capsulitis
23. Which of the following are most appropriate to utilize during the acute phase of adhesive capsulitis?
    A. Closed chain exercises
    B. Active full range of motion exercises
    C. Iontophoresis
    D. Eccentric resistance exercises
24. In the presence of adhesive capsulitis, with restricted glenohumeral motion, it is also essential to address which of the following during each phase of recovery?
    A. Active assistive full glenohumeral range of motion
    B. Scapular stabilization and motion exercises
    C. Plyometrics
    D. Closed kinetic chain exercises
    E. All of the above
25. Following a grade II A-C sprain, which of the following is the most common method of treatment?
    A. Surgery—ORIF
    B. Cast immobilization
    C. Shoulder harness and sling for 3 to 6 weeks
    D. Early active motion
26. During periods of immobilization following a grade II A-C sprain, which of the following can be prescribed?
    A. Isokinetic exercise
    B. Submaximal isometrics
    C. Eccentric exercise
    D. Closed chain exercise
    E. All of the above
27. Which of the following are associated injuries that occur in conjunction with scapular fractures?
    A. Other fractures
    B. Neurovascular injuries
    C. Glenohumeral dislocations
    D. Pneumothorax
    E. All of the above
28. Which of the following is a treatment for isolated fractures of the scapular body?
    A. ORIF procedure
    B. Immobilization for 8 to 12 weeks
    C. Immobilization for 2 to 3 weeks
    D. Complete bed rest for 6 weeks
29. Which of the following is the most common fracture of the scapula?
    A. Extraarticular glenoid neck
    B. Scapular body

C. Intraarticular glenoid neck
D. All glenoid neck fractures

30. If an intraarticular glenoid neck fracture is associated with glenohumeral instability, what is the treatment of choice?
    A. Ice, sling, and immobilization for 6 to 8 weeks
    B. Sling immobilization for 20 weeks
    C. Bed rest
    D. ORIF
31. Clavicular fractures occur commonly to:
    A. Women 20 to 30 years of age
    B. Men younger than 25 years of age
    C. Men between 30 and 45 years of age
    D. Women 25 years of age and younger
32. During immobilization of a proximal humerus fracture treated with an ORIF procedure, which of the following should be employed? (circle any that apply)
    A. Active shoulder flexion
    B. General conditioning program
    C. Active forward flexion
    D. Active hand, wrist, and elbow exercises for the arm of the affected shoulder
    E. Eccentric exercise
33. In an elderly person with a four-part proximal humerus fracture, which of the following is a potential significant clinical complication?
    A. Muscular atrophy
    B. Avascular necrosis
    C. Weakness
    D. Reduced ROM
34. With significant displaced four-part proximal humerus fractures in the elderly, which of the following may be most appropriate?
    A. ORIF procedure
    B. Immobilization for 6 to 10 weeks
    C. Prosthetic humeral head
    D. Fusion
35. Which of the following is an indication for a proximal humerus prosthesis or total shoulder arthroplasty?
    A. Avascular necrosis
    B. Rheumatoid arthritis
    C. Severe osteoarthritis
    D. Displaced Neer's four-part proximal humerus fractures
    E. All of the above
36. In terms of restoration of shoulder motion following a shoulder arthroplasty, if the rotator cuff is not repaired, postoperative shoulder abduction averages:
    A. 90°
    B. 110°

C. 143°
D. 160°

37. Those patients requiring rotator cuff repair in addition to shoulder arthroplasty may achieve an average abduction of:
A. 63°
B. 78°
C. 90°
D. 110°

38. By the end of the first postoperative week of rehabilitation following shoulder arthroplasty without rotator cuff repair, which of the following exercises should be are initiated?
A. Isokinetic exercises
B. Closed chain resistance
C. Codman's pendulum exercises
D. Eccentric loading

39. In general, when can light resistance exercises begin after shoulder arthroplasty?
A. End of the third week
B. By the sixth week
C. By the eighth week
D. By the twelfth week

SHORT ANSWER

40. In the following figure, identify the pathology and the structures involved.

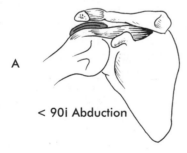

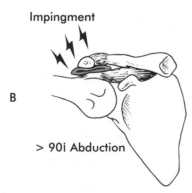

41. In the following figure, identify the lesion.

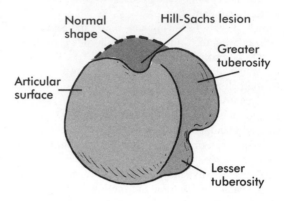

42. What does *TUBS* refer to in regard to shoulder instability?

43. What does *AMBRI* refer to in regard to shoulder instability?

44. In the following figure, identify the injury and the structures involved.

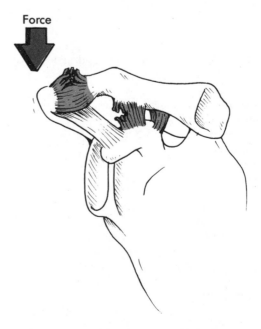

45. In the following figure, identify the injury and the structures involved.

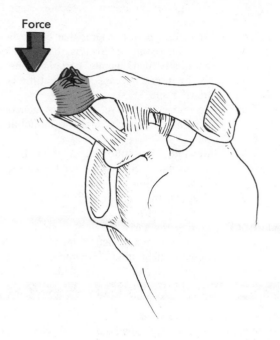

47. In the following figure, identify the specific type and location of this injury.

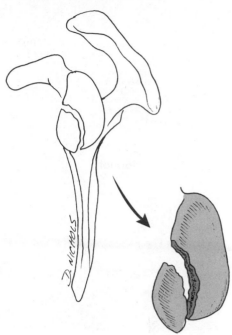

46. In the following figure, identify the technique or procedure and describe when it is used.

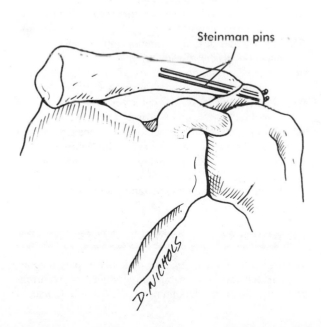

48. In the following figure, identify the device shown and describe for what it is used.

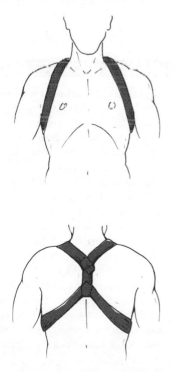

49. In the following figure, identify each of Neer's four-part proximal humerus fracture classification.

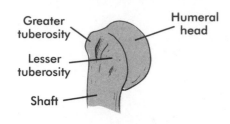

Greater tuberosity

Humeral head

Lesser tuberosity

Shaft

Normal

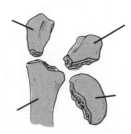

4 Part fracture

TRUE/FALSE

50. T or F   Secondary subacromial impingement is related to glenohumeral instability, which creates a reduced subacromial space, because the humeral head migrates upward and minimizes the area under the coracoacromial ligament.

51. T or F   Age-related arthritic changes and bony osteophyte formation have no effect on subacromial impingement of the shoulder.

52. T or F   Posterior shoulder dislocations occur more often than anterior dislocations.

53. T or F   It is not uncommon for rotator cuff tears to occur with shoulder dislocations.

54. T or F   During immobilization for anterior glenohumeral dislocation, it is necessary to provide range-of-motion and strengthening exercises for the hand, wrist, and elbow as well as of the affected shoulder.

55. T or F   Using the stair-stepper and treadmill is appropriate closed kinetic chain exercise to employ following shoulder dislocations during the minimum protection stage of recovery.

56. T or F   Transfer type procedures that utilize bone and soft tissue stabilization hardware occasionally demonstrate complications of the fixation devices as well as at the bone transfer site.

57. T or F   Secondary adhesive capsulitis generally occurs following trauma or immobilization.

58. T or F   Rehabilitation following a grade II A-C sprain must commence once the period of immobilization has ended.

59. T or F   Scapular fractures occur from indirect and insignificant trauma.

60. T or F   During the early recovery from direct rotator cuff repair, active muscle contractions of the deltoid are contraindicated.

ESSAY QUESTIONS

Answer on a separate sheet of paper.

61. Identify and describe methods, management, and rehabilitation for subacromial rotator cuff impingement.

62. Identify and describe methods of management and rehabilitation for tears of the rotator cuff.

63. Describe methods of management and rehabilitation for glenohumeral instability.

64. Discuss methods of management and rehabilitation for adhesive capsulitis.

65. Identify and describe common injuries of the acromioclavicular (A-C) joint.

66. Describe common methods of management and rehabilitation for injuries of the A-C joint.

67. Identify and describe common fractures of the scapula, clavicle, and proximal humerus.

68. Outline and describe methods of management and rehabilitation of fractures about the shoulder.

69. Describe methods of management and rehabilitation following shoulder arthroplasty.

70. Describe common mobilization techniques for the shoulder.

CRITICAL THINKING APPLICATION

As a role-playing activity, one student will play the part of a patient with a postoperative repair of recurrent traumatic anterior glenohumeral dislocation (coracoid transfer), while another student will play the role of a practicing PTA. For the "PTA": Based on your knowledge and understanding of bone and soft tissue healing, instruct the patient and demonstrate for a comprehensive initial postoperative care program. Is immobilization required? For how long? Why is this necessary? Specifically instruct your patient in the use of agents he or she can use at home for pain and swelling management. Discuss the rationale for the use of other agents you might use in the clinic for pain and swelling reduction. Which precautions would you outline for your patient? Clearly identify these and demonstrate. Which specific motion activities would you recommend? Have the patient demonstrate the correct performance of these exercises. What specific muscle contraction types are employed while the patient is immobilized? Describe these in detail and then have the patient demonstrate. List and demonstrate exercises for all other noninvolved joints that are appropriate. Thoroughly describe the rationale for scapulothoracic stability and strength related to this case. Have the patient demonstrate the correct performance of all scapulothoracic exercises you would recommend.

During the minimal protection phase, what role does eccentric loading play in the rehabilitation of anterior glenohumeral instability? Are closed kinetic chain proprioception exercises encouraged for this case? If so, describe three examples and have your patient demonstrate.

CHAPTER 17

Orthopedic Management of the Elbow

MULTIPLE CHOICE

1. Lateral epicondylitis is caused by:
   A. Acute direct trauma
   B. Concentric contraction of wrist flexors
   C. Overuse, repetitive motion disorder, cumulative trauma
   D. Eccentric loading of the biceps
   E. All of the above

2. Which of the following describe(s) the muscles of the common wrist extensor origin? (circle any that apply)
   A. Biceps brachii
   B. Extensor carpi radialis longus
   C. Extensor carpi radialis brevis
   D. Extensor digitorum
   E. Brachio radialis

3. Which of the following is not advocated during the early recovery phase of rehabilitation for lateral epicondylitis?

A. Ice
B. Phonophoresis
C. Functional activities
D. NSAIDs

4. Lateral epicondylitis occurs at what ratio to medial epicondylitis?
   A. 2:1
   B. 1:1
   C. 7:1
   D. 4:1

5. Which muscles make up the common flexor tendon of the medial epicondyle? (circle any that apply)
   A. Pronator teres
   B. Flexor carpi radialis
   C. Brachioradialis
   D. Flexor carpi ulnaris
   E. Biceps brachii

6. Supracondylar fractures occur most often to:
   A. Adults 25 to 40 years of age
   B. Older adults 55 to 75 years of age
   C. Younger women 20 to 30 years of age
   D. Children

7. Which of the following describes the types of supracondylar fractures?
   A. Type II
   B. Extension type
   C. Type I
   D. Flexion type
   E. All of the above

8. What is the most common treatment for supracondylar fractures?
   A. ORIF
   B. Rigid cast immobilization for 8 to 10 weeks
   C. Closed reduction and immobilization for 4 to 6 weeks
   D. Early active motion

9. Which of the following is considered the most significant complication following supracondylar fracture?
   A. Joint contracture
   B. Malunion
   C. Vascular compromise
   D. Nonunion
10. Which of the following is not a symptom of vascular obstruction following supracondylar fracture?
    A. Paresthesia
    B. Pain in forearm muscles
    C. Crepitus at fracture site
    D. Painful and reduced finger motion
11. A type I nondisplaced intercondylar fracture is treated with
    A. ORIF
    B. Active motion
    C. Immobilization for approximately 3 weeks
    D. Passive motion
12. Because of general bone quality (osteoporosis), which of the following can be used for treatment in an elderly patient with a type IV intercondylar fracture?
    A. ORIF
    B. "Bag of bones" procedure
    C. Early active motion
    D. Fusion
13. What is the average normal carrying angle for males?
    A. 15°
    B. 8°
    C. 10°
    D. 5°
14. What is the normal carrying angle for females?
    A. 13°
    B. 20°
    C. 10°
    D. 8°
15. Radial head fractures are generally classified into four types. Type I is defined as:
    A. Any radial head fracture with elbow dislocation
    B. A comminuted fracture
    C. A nondisplaced fracture
    D. A marginal fracture with displacement
16. Treatment of type I radial head fractures involves
    A. An ORIF procedure
    B. Immobilization for up to 4 weeks
    C. An excision
    D. Active motion
17. Type II radial head fractures are always treated with (circle any that apply)
    A. ORIF
    B. Immobilization

C. Excision
D. Fusion
E. Closed kinetic chain resistance
18. Which motion is most commonly affected (restricted) after radial head fractures? (circle any that apply)
    A. Flexion of the elbow
    B. Extension of the elbow
    C. Supination
    D. Pronation
    E. Radial deviation
19. Nondisplaced olecranon fractures are generally treated with
    A. ORIF
    B. Percutaneous pinning
    C. Immobilization for up to 8 weeks
    D. Excision
20. It is clinically important that flexion of the elbow, following nondisplaced olecranon fractures not exceed _____ for the first 6 to 8 weeks following injury.
    A. 45°
    B. 30°
    C. 90°
    D. 15°
21. For secure bone healing to occur, active elbow flexion past 90° and resistance exercises for elbow extension following olecranon fractures must be deferred for how many weeks following injury?
    A. 3 to 6 weeks
    B. 12 weeks or longer
    C. 8 weeks
    D. 3 to 4 weeks
22. What percentage of elbow dislocations are anterior?
    A. 10%
    B. 15%
    C. 1% to 2%
    D. 7%
23. Which of the following represents structures that can be injured as a result of elbow dislocation?
    A. Ulnar nerve
    B. Radial nerve
    C. Brachial artery
    D. Median nerve
    E. All of the above
24. Isolated posterior elbow dislocations are managed by:
    A. Immobilization in an extension
    B. ORIF
    C. Fusion
    D. Immobilization in flexion
25. Early active motion can usually begin after the first week following immobilization for a dislocated

elbow; however, passive stretching is related to the development of:

A. Flexion contractures
B. Vascular injury
C. Myositis ossificans
D. Extension contractures

26. What is the most common complication following elbow dislocation?
A. Myositis ossificans
B. Volkmann's ischemic contracture
C. Loss of elbow extension
D. Neurovascular compromise

27. Which of the following is the most common fracture that occurs with elbow dislocation?
A. Supracondylar fractures
B. Radial head fractures
C. Radius fractures
D. Ulnar fractures

SHORT ANSWER

28. In the following figure, identify the injury, mechanism of injury, and structure involved.

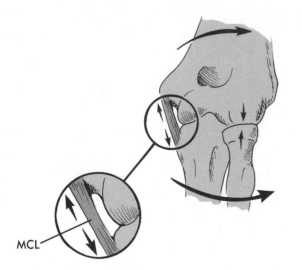

29. Name the most common type of supracondylar fracture.

30. In the following figure, identify the fracture type:

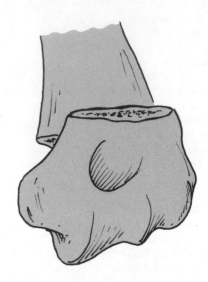

31. In the following figure, identify the general fracture, label the structure(s) that may be compromised, and identify the potential injury that may ensue.

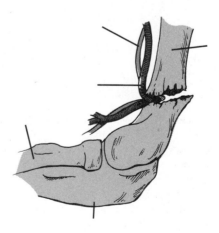

32. In the figure on the following page, identify the type and classification of fracture:

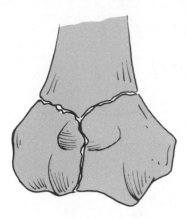

33. What is the most common direction of elbow dislocation?

TRUE/FALSE

34. T or F   In severe cases of "tennis elbow," the use of a wrist cock-up splint is advocated for the management of inflamed wrist extensor tendons.

35. T or F   During the subacute recovery phase of rehabilitation for lateral epicondylitis, initial instruction for patients to perform forearm pronation and supination must include the use of a hammer while holding the end of the shaft away from the head of the hammer.

36. T or F   Medial valgus stress overload is synonymous with medial epicondylitis.

37. T or F   The signs and symptoms of ischemic obstruction are always immediately evident following injury.

38. T or F   Passive stretching is advocated during the early recovery phase of healing following supracondylar fractures.

39. T or F   A type IV intercondylar fracture, which is severely comminuted with significant separation, is always treated with an ORIF procedure.

40. T or F   It is not uncommon for some patients to be left with some residual loss of motion following intercondylar fractures.

41. T or F   After excision of the radial head in type IV comminuted fractures, the radial shaft may migrate and cause pain at the distal radioulnar joint.

42. T or F   Displaced or comminuted fractures of the olecranon can be treated with an ORIF procedure or in cases of severely comminuted fractures; excision of as much as 80% of the olecranon.

43. T or F   With the exception of the shoulder, the elbow is the most frequently dislocated joint in the body.

ESSAY QUESTIONS

Answer on a separate sheet of paper.

44. Identify and describe common overuse, soft tissue injuries of the elbow.

45. Discuss common methods of management and rehabilitation of overuse, soft tissue injuries of the elbow.

46. Identify and describe intercondylar fractures, radial head fractures, olecranon fractures, and fracture-dislocations of the elbow.

47. Describe methods of management and rehabilitation of various fractures and fracture-dislocations of the elbow.

48. Describe common mobilization techniques for the elbow.

CRITICAL THINKING APPLICATION

Develop two case studies, one concerning a patient with a diagnosis of lateral epicondylitis, the other an elderly female with a type IV severely comminuted intercondylar fracture. In each case, outline and describe a comprehensive critical pathway (criterion-based rehabilitation program) concerning pain and swelling management, restoration of motion, muscle contraction types, cardiovascular fitness, general physical conditioning and open- and closed-chain proprioception activities. Your progressive recommendations should parallel the stages of bone and soft tissue healing and should be organized within the maximum protection phase, moderate protection phase, and minimal protection phase of recovery. What role does eccentric loading play in the recovery of lateral epicondylitis? What ADL activities would need to be modified with lateral epicondylitis?

Which significant vascular compromise is recognized with a supracondylar fracture? Describe which structures can be affected with this complication.

For an elderly person with osteoporosis, which method of stabilization would be most appropriate with a type IV comminuted intercondylar fracture? Which exercises can be employed during the period of immobilization?

Orthopedic Management of the Wrist and Hand

Carpal tunnel syndrome
Compression neuropathy
Nerve entrapment
De Quervain's tenosynovitis
Cumulative trauma disorder
Colles' fracture
Smith's fracture
Dinner fork deformity
Scaphoid fracture
Anatomic snuffbox
Avascular necrosis (AVN)
Nonunion
Skier's thumb
Boxer's fracture
Fighter's fracture
Bennett's fracture
Dupuytren's contracture
Mallet finger
Boutonniere deformity
Flexor tendon
Reflex sympathetic dystrophy (RSD)

MULTIPLE CHOICE

1. Which of the following is a clinical symptom of carpal tunnel syndrome?
   A. Pain
   B. Numbness
   C. Weakness
   D. Tingling
   E. All of the above

2. Carpal tunnel syndrome is considered: (circle any that apply)
   A. An acute traumatic injury
   B. A repetitive motion disorder
   C. An overuse injury
   D. A cumulative trauma injury
   E. Rare

3. After diagnosis, which of the following may have the greatest effect on reducing symptoms of carpal tunnel syndrome in the years ahead?
   A. Strengthening
   B. Stretching
   C. Identifying and modifying ADL and occupational risks
   D. Bracing

4. If a surgical release is performed for carpal tunnel syndrome (cutting of the transverse carpal ligament, thereby, decompressing the neurovascular tissues underneath), how long is the affected wrist immobilized?
   A. 6 to 8 weeks
   B. 3 to 5 weeks
   C. 2 to 14 days
   D. 8 to 10 weeks

5. Which of the following is(are) treatment for de Quervain's tenosynovitis? (circle any that apply)
   A. Wrist and thumb immobilized
   B. Corticosteroid injection
   C. Surgical decompression
   D. Excision of the radial styloid
   E. Tendon release

6. Ligament sprains of the wrist, without carpal instability, are managed with:
   A. Percutaneous pinning
   B. Immobilization
   C. ORIF

D. Direct surgical repair of torn ligaments
E. All of the above

7. Ligament sprains of the wrist with resultant carpal instability can be treated with: (circle any that apply)
A. ORIF
B. Closed reduction with percutaneous pinning
C. Cast immobilization
D. Fusion of carpals
E. Early active full ROM

8. A Colles' fracture affects primarily which of the following?
A. Teenage males
B. Elderly males
C. Middle-age and elderly females
D. Young females

9. If a Colles' fracture is minimally displaced and stable, the method of treatment is usually:
A. Percutaneous pinning
B. ORIF
C. Closed reduction with rigid immobilization
D. Sling immobilization

10. Which of the following are identified as possible complications following Colles' fractures?
A. Nonunion
B. Tendon adhesions
C. Median nerve compression
D. Reflex sympathetic dystrophy
E. All of the above

11. Avulsion fractures of the ulnar styloid can occur in _____ of unstable distal radius fractures.
A. 10%
B. 90%
C. 50%
D. 60%

12. Which of the following is a major concern following proximal pole fractures of the scaphoid?
A. Muscular weakness
B. Avascular necrosis
C. Arthrofibrosis
D. Wrist flexion contracture
E. All of the above

13. Where is pain most clinically significant in the presence of a scaphoid fracture?
A. Volar aspect of the wrist (diffuse)
B. Dorsal aspect of the wrist (diffuse)
C. Anatomic "snuffbox"
D. Ulnar styloid

14. In cases where the scaphoid fracture is nondisplaced and stable, the treatment is usually with closed reduction and rigid cast immobilization for approxi-

mately 6 weeks. However, fractures of the proximal pole require immobilization for:
A. 8 weeks
B. 12 to 24 weeks
C. 10 weeks
D. 9 to 11 weeks

15. If nonunion or avascular necrosis occurs following a proximal pole scaphoid fracture, which of the following can be employed to aid healing? (circle any that apply)
A. Bone grafts
B. Electrical stimulation
C. Vascular shunts
D. Closed kinetic chain exercises
E. Early active motion

16. Which of the following describe(s) the cornerstone of treatment for scaphoid fractures? (circle any that apply)
A. Early active motion
B. Fracture site protection
C. Closed kinetic chain exercises
D. Immobilization
E. Early proprioception exercises

17. In general, which of the following are indications that physicians should consider for an ORIF for metacarpal fractures?
A. Articular fractures
B. Unstable fractures
C. Bone loss
D. Open fractures
E. All of the above

18. A proliferative fibrodysplasia disease that affects the palmar fascia and leads to contractures is called:
A. De Quervain's disease
B. Volkmann's contracture
C. Dupuytren's contracture
D. Palmar fasciitis

19. Dupuytren's contracture affects mainly:
A. Women 20 to 40 years of age
B. Young males 25 years of age and younger
C. Males 40 years of age and older
D. Women 45 to 60 years of age

20. Treatment of Dupuytren's contracture is centered on:
A. Resolution of painful nodules
B. Correction of deformity and loss of function
C. Improving vascular supply to the palmar fascia
D. Increasing wrist flexion motion

21. Which of the following describes a clinically significant feature following fasciectomy for Dupuytren's contracture?
A. The sutures are left in place for only 7 to 10 days
B. The surgical incision is left open

C. There is significant sensory loss

D. Extreme pain is noted for many days

22. To restore function following surgery for Dupuytren's contracture, which of the following exercises is employed to enhance early motion?

    A. Finger flexion to distal palmar crease (active)

    B. Active PIP flexion

    C. Active abduction and adduction of the fingers

    D. Active finger extension

    E. All of the above

23. Which of the following are appropriate treatment measures for extensor tendon rupture or avulsion fracture of the fingers? (circle any that apply)

    A. DIP flexion with splinting

    B. Continuous splinting for 6 to 10 weeks

    C. Active extension

    D. DIP terminal extension with splinting

    E. ORIF

24. Which of the following is contraindicated following extensor tendon rupture or avulsion fracture?

    A. Active extension of the DIP between the sixth and eighth weeks

    B. Active flexion of the DIP to 20°

    C. Passive flexion of the DIP

    D. Passive extension of the DIP

25. In general, flexor tendon injuries and repairs are treated with:

    A. Rigid immobilization for 6 to 10 weeks

    B. Immobilization for 10 weeks or longer

    C. Early protected motion

    D. Immobilization for 4 to 6 weeks

26. Which of the following is characteristic of reflex sympathetic dystrophy?

    A. Edema

    B. Loss of function

    C. Pain

    D. Hyperesthesia

    E. All of the above

27. Which of the following are clinical symptoms of stage I RSD?

    A. Pale cyanosis

    B. Production of inelastic fibrous tissue

    C. Increased tissue atrophy

    D. Pain and edema, discoloration, and hyperhydrosis

28. The treatment of RSD is primarily focused on:

    A. Restoration of strength

    B. Improved motion

    C. Pain and swelling management

    D. Early return to functional activities

29. Which of the following is a measure that can be employed to manage pain and swelling with RSD? (circle any that apply)

    A. Ice

    B. Heat

    C. TENS, electrical stimulation

    D. Sympathetic nerve block injections

    E. Full active range of motion

30. Which of the following is(are) strictly avoided during each stage of recovery with RSD if pain is present? (circle any that apply)

    A. Splint applications

    B. Plyometrics

    C. Full range slow- and fast-speed isokinetic exercise

    D. Eccentric full-range isotonic exercise

    E. Thermal agents

SHORT ANSWER

31. Name the most common compression neuropathy of the wrist.

32. In the following figure, identify the injury and the tissues involved:

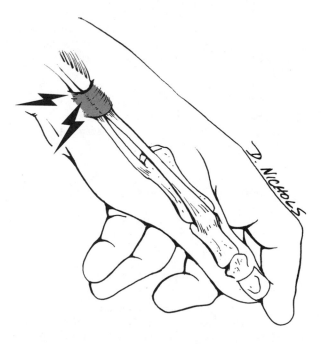

33. In the following figure, identify the injury and name
the common deformity:

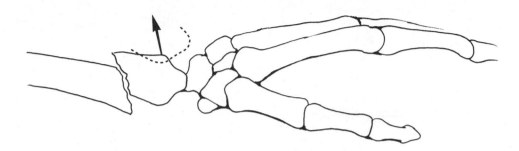

34. In the following figure, identify the injury and
describe the method of fixation:

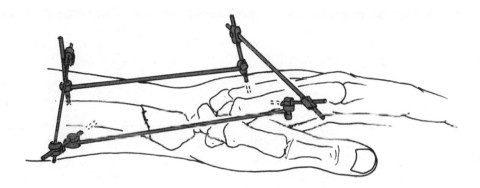

35. Name the injury in the following figure:

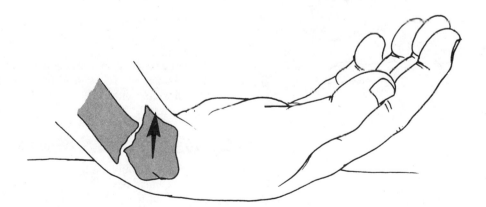

36. In the following figure, identify the injury and the structures involved. Also identify a common name for this injury:

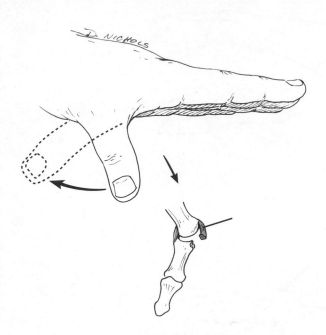

37. Identify the injury in the figure and give a common name that describes the injury:

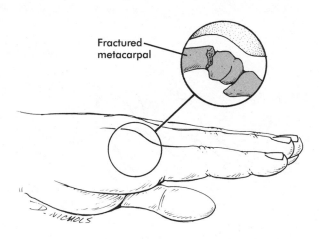

Fractured metacarpal

38. A fracture-subluxation of the proximal first metacarpal describes what type of fracture?

39. Identify the injuries or deformities in the following figures:

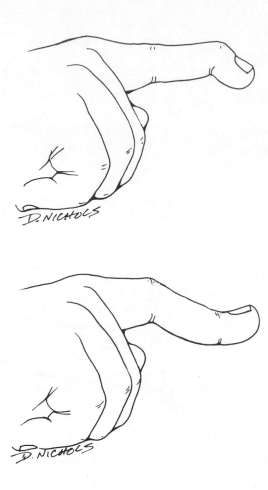

40. A rupture or avulsion fracture of the extensor tendon that results in a DIP joint flexion contracture is called _____ .

41. A rupture or stretch of the central extensor tendon at the proximal interphalangeal (PIP) joint that creates PIP flexion with DIP extension is called a _____ .

TRUE/FALSE

42. T or F   Generally, motions that produce repetitive ulnar deviations can create tenosynovitis at the first dorsal compartment of the wrist.

43. T or F   The stability of the wrist is primarily dependent on musculotendinous support as well as intracapsular ligaments.
44. T or F   A Colles' fracture is the most common of all fractures.
45. T or F   Distal ulnar fractures commonly occur as isolated injuries.
46. T or F   Scaphoid fractures are considered the most common fractures that occur to the carpal bones.
47. T or F   Although occasionally tender nodules are present, Dupuytren's contracture is commonly not painful.
48. T or F   If a 20° to 30° flexion contracture of the ulnar metacarpalphalangeal (MCP) joint results from Dupuytren's' contracture, then an open surgical procedure (fasciectomy or excision of the palmar fascia) should be performed.
49. T or F   There is usually a direct relationship between the severity of injury and the degree of pain experienced by persons suffering from RSD.
50. T or F   It is true that at no point in the course of recovery from RSD is aggressive active motion prescribed in the presence of pain.

ESSAY QUESTIONS

Answer on a separate sheet of paper.
51. Identify and describe common compression neuropathies of the wrist.
52. Discuss methods of management and rehabilitation of compression neuropathies of the wrist.
53. Identify and describe common ligament injuries of the wrist.
54. Describe and discuss methods of management and rehabilitation of ligament injuries of the wrist.
55. Describe methods of management and rehabilitation for distal radial and ulnar fractures.
56. Identify methods of management and rehabilitation for scaphoid fractures.
57. Identify and describe common metacarpal fractures and methods of management and rehabilitation.
58. Describe methods of management and rehabilitation of Dupuytren's contracture.
59. Identify and describe common extensor and flexor tendon injuries.
60. Discuss methods of management and rehabilitation of extensor tendon and flexor tendon injuries.
61. Identify methods of management and rehabilitation for reflex sympathetic dystrophy.
62. Describe common mobilization techniques for the wrist and hand.

CRITICAL THINKING APPLICATION

You are treating two patients, one with the diagnosis of carpal tunnel syndrome (nonoperative), the other with a stable, minimally displaced Colles' fracture. Based on your understanding of bone and soft tissue healing, develop a comprehensive critical pathway (criterion-based rehabilitation program) for each case in which you will recommend specific therapeutic interventions for pain and swelling management, restoration of motion, muscle contraction types, cardiovascular fitness, general physical conditioning, and closed-chain proprioception functional activities. Organize your outline so that the rehabilitation program you recommend parallels the phases of soft tissue and bone healing, which in turn coincides with the maximum protection phase, moderate protection phase, and minimum protection phase of recovery.

Which ergonomic and functional ADL modifications do you recommend for the patient with carpal tunnel syndrome? Which exercises and activities do you recommend for the patient with the Colles' fracture during periods of immobilization? Clearly note and identify complications which can occur following a Colles' fracture.

Answer Key

CHAPTER 1

Patient Supervision and Observation During Treatment

MULTIPLE CHOICE

1. F

SHORT ANSWER

2. See page 4 in textbook.
3. See page 4 in textbook.
4. Communication
5. Understanding, sensitivity, warmth, and reassurance
6. Listening
7. Open-end questions
8. Closed-end questions
9. See page 6 in textbook.
10. See page 6 in textbook.
11. Summary-type statements
12. See page 7 in textbook.
13. Dominance, submission, hostility, warmth
14.

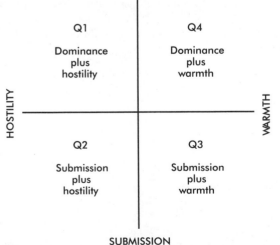

15. Q4
16. Appropriately friendly, attentive, responsive, involved, exploring, analytical, and task oriented (see page 8 in textbook)
17. See page 8 in textbook.
18. See page 9 in textbook.
19. Goniometric measurements (ROM); circumferential measurements (swelling, hypertrophy, atrophy); manual muscle testing; endurance; heart rate, blood pressure; respirations; balance; coordination

ESSAY QUESTIONS

20. See page 5 in textbook.
21. See page 6 in textbook.
22. See page 4 in textbook.
23. See page 6 in textbook.
24. See page 6 in textbook.
25. See page 8 in textbook.
26. See page 8 in textbook.
27. See page 8 in textbook.

CHAPTER 2

Flexibility

MULTIPLE CHOICE

1. C
2. B
3. E
4. C
5. D
6. C
7. C
8. C and D
9. D
10. B
11. D

SHORT ANSWER

12. Active
13. Static, ballistic, PNF
14. Golgi tendon organ (GTO)
15. Muscle spindle

TRUE/FALSE

16. T
17. F
18. T
19. T
20. T
21. F
22. F

ESSAY QUESTIONS

23. See page 12 in textbook.
24. See page 12 in textbook.
25. See page 12 in textbook.
26. See page 12 in textbook.
27. See page 13 in textbook.
28. See page 14 in textbook.
29. See page 17 in textbook.
30. See page 19 in textbook.
31. See page 20 in textbook.
32. See page 24 in textbook.

CHAPTER 3
Strength

MULTIPLE CHOICE

1. D
2. D
3. C and D
4. B
5. B, D, and E
6. D
7. E
8. A, C, and D
9. B, C, and D
10. A, B, and C
11. B, D, and E
12. B
13. C
14. C
15. B
16. C
17. D
18. C

19. C
20. D
21. C
22. D
23. C
24. E

SHORT ANSWER

25. Two
26. Oxidative
27. 1. Slow twitch (type I)
    2. Fast twitch (type II)
    3. Fast twitch (type II-A)
    4. Fast twitch (type II-AB)
    5. Fast twitch (type II-B)
28. Manual muscle testing, cable tensiometry, dynamometry, isotonic one-repetition maximum lift, isokinetics
29. 3. Concentrics
    2. Isometrics
    1. Eccentrics
30. 3. Eccentrics
    2. Isometrics
    1. Concentrics
31. Atrophy and hypertrophy
32. Specific Adaptions to Imposed Demands
33. Frequency, intensity, and duration
34. See page 37 in textbook.

TRUE/FALSE

35. T
36. F
37. F
38. F
39. T
40. F
41. F
42. F
43. T
44. F
45. T
46. F
47. F

ESSAY QUESTIONS

48. See page 29 in textbook.
49. See page 30 in textbook.
50. See page 30 in textbook.
51. See page 30 in textbook.
52. See page 32 in textbook.
53. See page 32 in textbook.
54. See page 33 in textbook.
55. See page 34 in textbook.

56. See page 35 in textbook.
57. See page 37 in textbook.
58. See page 37 in textbook.
59. See page 38 in textbook.
60. See page 40 in textbook.
61. See page 42 in textbook.
62. See page 45 in textbook.

CHAPTER 4
Endurance

MULTIPLE CHOICE

1. D
2. C
3. E
4. B and D
5. B
6. C
7. A
8. C
9. B
10. C
11. B and D
12. A, B, and C
13. B, C, and D

TRUE/FALSE

14. F

ESSAY QUESTIONS

15. See page 51 in textbook.
16. See page 51 in textbook.
17. See page 51 in textbook.
18. See page 52 in textbook.
19. See page 52 in textbook.
20. See page 53 in textbook.
21. See page 55 in textbook.
22. See page 56 in textbook.

CHAPTER 5
Balance and Coordination

MULTIPLE CHOICE

1. E
2. C
3. A

4. C
5. C
6. B
7. E
8. E
9. A, B, and C

SHORT ANSWER

10. Provide manual external resistance; ask the patient to close his or her eyes.
11. Single-leg stance test (SLST)
12. 1. Sitting balance—eyes open
    2. Standing—weight shifting
    3. Double-leg standing—eyes closed
    4. Single-leg standing—eyes closed
    5. Single-leg standing—eyes closed with manual resistance
13. See page 63 in textbook.

TRUE/FALSE

14. T
15. F
16. F
17. T
18. T
19. T
20. T
21. F

ESSAY QUESTIONS

22. See page 58 in textbook.
23. See page 58 in textbook.
24. See page 59 in textbook.
25. See page 59 in textbook.
26. See page 60 in textbook.
27. See page 60 in textbook.
28. See page 63 in textbook.

CHAPTER 6
Ligament Healing

MULTIPLE CHOICE

1. B
2. A
3. D
4. D
5. A
6. B
7. D

8. C and D
9. A and B
10. B and D
11. C
12. C
13. E
14. B, C, D, and E

SHORT ANSWER

15. Phase I: inflammatory response
    Phase II: repair
    Phase III: remodeling
16. Redness, swelling, pain, heat, loss of function
17. Repair phase
18. Contact, controlled stress, excessive forces
19. See page 77 in textbook.

TRUE/FALSE

20. F
21. F
22. F
23. F
24. F
25. T

ESSAY QUESTIONS

26. See page 67 in textbook.
27. See page 67 in textbook.
28. See page 67 in textbook.
29. See page 74 in textbook.
30. See page 75 in textbook.
31. See page 76 in textbook.

CHAPTER 7
Bone Healing

MULTIPLE CHOICE

1. B, C, and D
2. C
3. D
4. D
5. E
6. B, C, and D
7. A, C, and D
8. C
9. D
10. C and D
11. C
12. A and D

13. A and C
14. C
15. A and B
16. E
17. E
18. E

SHORT ANSWER

19. Internal and external fixation
20. Pain, crepitus, swelling

TRUE/FALSE

21. F
22. T
23. T

ESSAY QUESTIONS

24. See page 82 in textbook.
25. See page 81 in textbook.
26. See page 82 in textbook.
27. See page 83 in textbook.
28. See page 84 in textbook.
29. See page 84 in textbook.
30. See page 81 in textbook.
31. See page 81 in textbook.
32. See page 82 in textbook.
33. See page 82 in textbook.
34. See page 82 in textbook.
35. See page 85 in textbook.
36. See page 86 in textbook.

CHAPTER 8
Cartilage Healing

MULTIPLE CHOICE

1. B
2. E
3. A, B, D, and E
4. C and D
5. C and D
6. B, C, and D
7. E
8. B
9. E
10. C
11. C
12. A and C
13. A, C, D, and E
14. A and B

SHORT ANSWER

15. Total meniscectomy, subtotal meniscectomy, meniscal repair
16. Traumatic or degenerative

TRUE/FALSE

17. T
18. T
19. F
20. F
21. F
22. F
23. T

ESSAY QUESTIONS

24. See page 89 in textbook.
25. See page 89 in textbook.
26. See page 89 in textbook.
27. See page 90 in textbook.
28. See page 91 in textbook.
29. See page 91 in textbook.
30. See page 91 in textbook.
31. See page 92 in textbook.

CHAPTER 9

Muscle and Tendon Healing

MULTIPLE CHOICE

1. D
2. C and D
3. C
4. A
5. B
6. D
7. A, B, and C
8. C
9. D
10. C and D
11. C
12. B
13. C

SHORT ANSWER

14. Indirect
15. Direct

TRUE/FALSE

16. T
17. T
18. T
19. T
20. T
21. F

ESSAY QUESTIONS

22. See page 95 in textbook.
23. See page 95 in textbook.
24. See page 95 in textbook.
25. See page 95 in textbook.
26. See page 95 in textbook.
27. See page 96 in textbook.
28. See page 97 in textbook.
29. See page 97 in textbook.
30. See page 98 in textbook.
31. See page 98 in textbook.

CHAPTER 10

Fundamentals of Gait

MULTIPLE CHOICE

1. D
2. B
3. B
4. B
5. D
6. A
7. C
8. C
9. C
10. B
11. C
12. B
13. B
14. A
15. C
16. E
17. B
18. D
19. C
20. A
21. D
22. C
23. D
24. C
25. C

SHORT ANSWER

26. Step length
27. Stance phase, swing phase
28. Heel strike, foot flat, midstance, heel off, toe off
29. Acceleration, midswing, deceleration
30. Shock absorption
31. Uninvolved side

TRUE/FALSE

32. T
33. F
34. T

ESSAY QUESTIONS

35. See page 104 in textbook.
36. See page 107 in textbook.
37. See page 107 in textbook.
38. See page 107 in textbook.
39. See page 108 in textbook.
40. See page 109 in textbook.
41. See page 110 in textbook.

21. C
22. B, D, and E
23. E

SHORT ANSWER

24. Opposite
25. Same

TRUE/FALSE

26. F
27. T
28. T
29. F

ESSAY QUESTIONS

30. See page 112 in textbook.
31. See page 112 in textbook.
32. See page 112 in textbook.
33. See page 113 in textbook.
34. See page 114 in textbook.
35. See page 116 in textbook.
36. See page 116 in textbook.
37. See page 116 in textbook.

CHAPTER 11

Concepts of Joint Mobilization

MULTIPLE CHOICE

1. C
2. C, D, and E
3. B
4. C and D
5. C
6. B
7. A
8. B
9. C
10. C
11. B
12. A
13. D
14. B
15. C
16. B
17. C
18. A
19. B
20. A, C, and D

CHAPTER 12

Orthopedic Management of the Ankle, Foot, and Toes

MULTIPLE CHOICE

1. C
2. C
3. B
4. E
5. B
6. C
7. B
8. D
9. D
10. A
11. B
12. C
13. B, C, D, and E
14. C
15. C
16. D
17. B
18. C and D
19. C

20. C and E
21. C and D
22. A
23. D
24. D
25. C
26. C
27. B
28. B
29. E
30. D
31. B, C, and D
32. C
33. A and B
34. E
35. B
36. E
37. C
38. D
39. C
40. D
41. B
42. A and C
43. B
44. C
45. E
46. E
47. B
48. A, B, D, and E
49. A and C
50. C

SHORT ANSWER

51. Mechanical and functional
52. Anterior talofibular, fibulocalcaneal, posterior talofibular
53. See page 144 in textbook.
54. A. Mallet toe

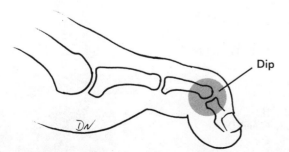

B. Claw toe

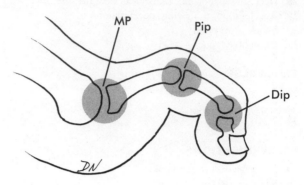

C. Hammer toe

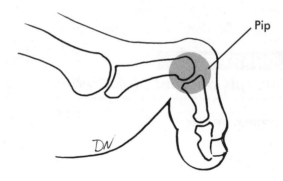

TRUE/FALSE

55. F
56. T
57. T
58. F
59. F
60. T
61. T
62. T
63. F
64. T
65. T
66. F

ESSAY QUESTIONS

67. See page 122 in textbook.
68. See page 124 in textbook.
69. See page 129 in textbook.
70. See page 129 in textbook.
71. See page 135 in textbook.
72. See page 137 in textbook.
73. See page 144 in textbook.
74. See page 145 in textbook.

CHAPTER 13

Orthopedic Management of the Knee

MULTIPLE CHOICE

1. B and D
2. C
3. C
4. D
5. C
6. D
7. C
8. D
9. B
10. C
11. B and C
12. A, B, C, and D
13. B
14. A and B
15. C
16. C
17. C, D, and E
18. A, B, and E
19. A and C
20. B, C, and D
21. A
22. C
23. C
24. B
25. C
26. B
27. A, B, and D
28. B
29. B
30. B
31. B
32. D
33. C
34. C
35. A, B, and E
36. A, D, and E
37. B
38. A
39. B
40. B and D
41. C
42. B
43. C
44. C
45. C
46. B, C, and D
47. A, B, C, and E
48. E
49. B
50. C
51. E
52. A, B, and C
53. C
54. C
55. D
56. E
57. A, B, and C
58. B and C
59. A
60. E
61. C and D
62. A
63. B
64. A
65. B
66. D

SHORT ANSWER

67. ACL tear
68. Ligament is PCL; exam is anterior drawer test
69. Mechanism of injury is valgus force; torn structure is MCL sprain
70. A. Bucket handle
    B. Parrot break
    C. Longitudinal
71. A. Red-on-white zone
    B. White-on-white zone
    C. Red-on-red zone
72. A. Patella alta
    B. Normal
    C. Patella baja
73. Patellar mobility, active quad strengthening exercises, active knee flexion
74. Transverse patella fracture; tension band wire and cerclage wire
75. Constrained, nonconstrained

TRUE/FALSE

76. T
77. F

78. F
79. F
80. F
81. F
82. T
83. T
84. F
85. F
86. T
87. T
88. F
89. T
90. F
91. F
92. F
93. T
94. F

ESSAY QUESTIONS

95. See page 150 in textbook.
96. See page 153 in textbook.
97. See page 165 in textbook.
98. See page 166 in textbook.
99. See page 169 in textbook.
100. See page 171 in textbook.
101. See page 175 in textbook.
102. See page 176 in textbook.
103. See page 180 in textbook.
104. See page 184 in textbook.

CHAPTER 14

Orthopedic Management of the Hip and Pelvis

MULTIPLE CHOICE

1. A and C
2. C
3. B and D
4. C
5. C
6. B
7. B
8. C
9. E
10. C
11. B
12. D
13. A, C, and D
14. C, D, and E

15. C
16. A and C
17. C
18. C
19. B, C, and D
20. C
21. C
22. B, C, and E

SHORT ANSWER

23. Subtrochanteric hip fracture
24. Femoral neck fracture
25. Intertrochanteric hip fracture
26. Greater trochanteric bursitis
27. Iliopectineal bursitis
28. Ischial bursitis
29.

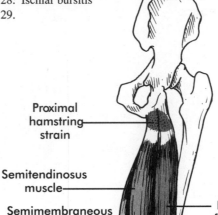

Proximal hamstring strain

Semitendinosus muscle

Semimembraneous muscle

Biceps femoris muscle

30. Avulsion fracture of iliac crest

TRUE/FALSE

31. T
32. T
33. F
34. T

35. T
36. T
37. T
38. F
39. T
40. F

ESSAY QUESTIONS

41. See page 189 in textbook.
42. See page 192 in textbook.
43. See page 198 in textbook.
44. See page 201 in textbook.
45. See page 202 in textbook.
46. See page 204 in textbook.
47. See page 207 in textbook.
48. See page 209 in textbook.

CHAPTER 15

Orthopedic Management of the Lumbar, Thoracic, and Cervical Spine

MULTIPLE CHOICE

1. D
2. A
3. C
4. A, C, D, and E
5. E
6. E
7. B, C, and D
8. C
9. C
10. D
11. C
12. E
13. E
14. A
15. A, B, and D
16. D
17. E
18. B, C, and D
19. E
20. D
21. A
22. C
23. A
24. D
25. B

26. C
27. C
28. A
29. C
30. B
31. B
32. E
33. C
34. E
35. E
36. C
37. E
38. B, C, and D
39. C
40. C
41. B and D
42. C
43. E
44. C

SHORT ANSWER

45. 100%—standing
    75%—sidelying
    35%—supine (knees flexed)
    25%—supine
    275%—bending forward
46. Load, lever, lordosis, legs, and lungs
47. Disc protrusion
48. Sequestrated disc

TRUE/FALSE

49. T
50. T
51. F
52. F
53. F
54. T
55. F
56. T
57. T
58. F
59. T
60. F
61. F

ESSAY QUESTIONS

62. See page 212 in textbook.
63. See page 214 in textbook.
64. See page 216 in textbook.
65. See page 217 in textbook.
66. See page 221 in textbook.
67. See page 223 in textbook.

68. See page 215 in textbook.
69. See page 230 in textbook.
70. See page 231 in textbook.
71. See page 226 in textbook.
72. See page 227 in textbook.
73. See page 228 in textbook.
74. See page 229 in textbook.
75. See page 232 in textbook.
76. See page 232 in textbook.
77. See page 236 in textbook.

CHAPTER 16

Orthopedic Management of the Shoulder

MULTIPLE CHOICE

1. C
2. C
3. B, C, and D
4. B, D, and E
5. A, B, and D
6. B and D
7. A
8. B
9. A, B, and D
10. A
11. A, C, and D
12. C
13. B
14. C
15. C
16. C
17. C
18. A, C, and D
19. E
20. C
21. C and D
22. B
23. C
24. B
25. C
26. B
27. E
28. C
29. B
30. D
31. B
32. B and D
33. B
34. C
35. E
36. C
37. A
38. C
39. B

SHORT ANSWER

40. Subacromial rotator cuff impingement; supraspinatus tendon
41. Hill-Sachs lesion
42. Traumatic unidirectional instability and Bankart lesion that frequently requires surgery
43. Atraumatic multidirectional bilateral instability; responds to rehabilitation; occasionally patients require inferior capsular shift
44. Grade II A-C sprain; rupture of A-C ligament plus partial tear of coracoacromial ligament
45. Grade I A-C sprain; partial tear of A-C ligament
46. Pin insertion to stabilize grade III A-C sprain
47. Intraarticular fracture of glenoid
48. Figure-of-eight bandage; used for clavicle fracture
49.

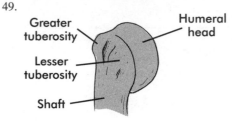

Normal

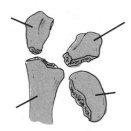

4 Part fracture

TRUE/FALSE

50. T
51. F
52. F

53. T
54. T
55. T
56. T
57. T
58. F
59. F
60. T

ESSAY QUESTIONS

61. See page 244 in textbook.
62. See page 247 in textbook.
63. See page 250 in textbook.
64. See page 257 in textbook.
65. See page 258 in textbook.
66. See page 259 in textbook.
67. See page 261 in textbook.
68. See page 261 in textbook.
69. See page 264 in textbook.
70. See page 265 in textbook.

CHAPTER 17

Orthopedic Management of the Elbow

MULTIPLE CHOICE

1. C
2. B, C, and D
3. C
4. C
5. A, B, and D
6. D
7. E
8. C
9. C
10. C
11. C
12. B
13. C
14. A
15. C
16. B
17. A and C
18. C and D
19. C
20. C
21. C
22. C
23. E

24. D
25. C
26. C
27. B

SHORT ANSWER

28. Medial valgus stress; repetitive valgus stress; medial collateral ligament
29. Type I—extension
30. Type II—flexion type supracondylar fracture
31. Supracondylar fracture; brachial artery; Volkmann's ischemic contracture
32. Type I—intercondylar nondisplaced fracture
33. Posterior dislocations

TRUE/FALSE

34. T
35. F
36. F
37. F
38. F
39. F
40. T
41. T
42. T
43. T

ESSAY QUESTIONS

44. See page 270 in textbook.
45. See page 270 in textbook.
46. See page 275 in textbook.
47. See page 276 in textbook.
48. See page 281 in textbook.

CHAPTER 18

Orthopedic Management of the Wrist and Hand

MULTIPLE CHOICE

1. E
2. B, C, and D
3. C
4. C
5. A, B, C
6. B
7. A, B, C
8. C
9. C

10. E
11. B
12. B
13. C
14. B
15. A and B
16. B and D
17. E
18. C
19. C
20. B
21. B
22. E
23. B, C, and D
24. C
25. C
26. E
27. D
28. C
29. B, C, and D
30. B, C, and D

SHORT ANSWER

31. Carpal tunnel syndrome
32. de Quervain's tenosynovitis; abductor pollicis longus, extensor pollicis brevis
33. Colles' fracture; dinner fork deformity
34. Colles' comminuted fracture; external fixator
35. Smith fracture
36. Valgus hyperextension of the thumb; sprain of ulnar collateral ligament; gamekeeper's thumb, skier's thumb
37. Fractured metacarpal; boxer's fracture, fighter's fracture
38. Bennett's fracture
39. Mallet finger

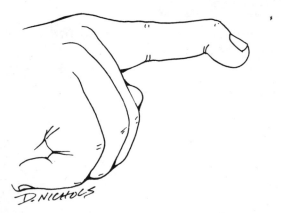

Boutonniere deformity

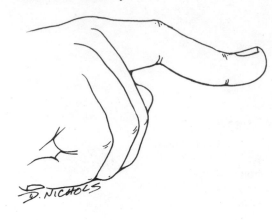

40. Mallet finger
41. Boutonniere deformity

TRUE/FALSE

42. T
43. F
44. T
45. F
46. T
47. T
48. T
49. F
50. T

ESSAY QUESTIONS

51. See page 284 in textbook.
52. See page 284 in textbook.
53. See page 286 in textbook.
54. See page 286 in textbook.
55. See page 287 in textbook.
56. See page 289 in textbook.
57. See page 291 in textbook.
58. See page 292 in textbook.
59. See page 293 in textbook.
60. See page 294 in textbook.
61. See page 295 in textbook.
62. See page 296 in textbook.